Life

On The

Triad

Meal Plan And Recipe Companion
To *The Weight Loss Triad*

Dr. Thomas L. Halton

Published by
Fitness Plus

First Edition

Published by Fitness Plus
Boston, MA

ISBN 978-0-988-2314-1-2

Table of Contents

Disclaimer

This book is intended for informational and educational purposes only. It is not meant to provide counseling, nor to provide medical advice. Always be sure to consult with your physician before starting any exercise program.

Chapter #1
Introduction

Losing weight is tough for a lot of reasons. First of all, everything about our modern American society promotes sedentary living and unhealthy eating. Food companies and restaurant chains spend millions of dollars each year researching the proper combinations of fat, sugar, and salt to quite literally addict you to their food. These restaurants aren't happy if you come back once every few weeks; they want your visit to be a daily occurrence. Let me tell you—they are good at what they do. Junk food is extremely addicting.

Very few of us work with our hands or on our feet. Sedentary work habits, combined with cars, elevators, and escalators have removed much of the built in physical activity from our lives. Most of us start out really active when we are little. Many of us play sports in grammar school, junior high, and high school. A few of us are lucky and good enough to play college sports. After that, physical activity largely leaves our lives unless we make a very deliberate effort to be active. Very few of us make this effort.

This combination of our eating habits and our sedentary lifestyles has a nasty effect on our weight and health. The default for the typical American nowadays is to become overweight some time in their late 20's and early 30's, obese in their 40's, and then pretty sick from their 50's onward to an early exit from this wonderful world.

Our diet and exercise habits are naturally a huge part of this problem, but they are not the whole story. A fundamental lack of knowledge is just as important. Nutrition information is extremely confusing to most people. In many cases, researchers, the government, your doctor, and the media will all have a different opinion about how you should be eating. Who do you listen to? Most bestselling diet books are written by people who have never even cracked a basic nutrition textbook once in their life. I know that in America we are totally obsessed with celebrities, but should they really be telling us how to eat to improve our health?

I honestly believe that most people who fail at weight loss didn't have the knowledge that they needed to succeed. There is a body of nutrition research out there that is pretty impressive, but also largely unknown, even by most doctors and dieticians. When you truly understand what it takes to lose weight, your battle is half won.

Hopefully we can sort out all of this misinform-ation together. After reading this book, I'm confident that you'll learn what you have to do to attain your weight loss goals. Here's the first thing you must realize: *Weight loss is not easy or fast, and fad diets don't work.* Changing your weight takes continued effort and daily focus on your diet, exercise, and lifestyle habits. Anyone who tells you otherwise is wrong.

This book is a follow up to my first book, *The Weight Loss Triad.* In *The Weight Loss Triad,* I outlined the three major components of successful, long term weight loss. The three areas are: 1) A blood sugar stabilizing diet, 2) The right type and amount of cardiovascular exercise, and 3) Resistance training. The program I developed is a combination of my graduate education and research, as well as my 15 years of working with weight loss clients. It is both research based and highly practical.

I will be the first to tell you that it is not always easy, but I'll also be the first to tell you that it really works, and nothing less will get the job done. After all of these years, I'm still amazed at how this program can change lives. Nothing puts a smile on my face as much as getting an email from a reader of *The Weight Loss Triad* who is thanking me for helping them to finally get control of their weight and improve their health.

For those of you who are not familiar with my first book, I'd like to start out with a little bit about my background. My name is Thomas L Halton. I recently graduated Harvard University with a Doctor of Science in Nutritional Epidemiology. This is a fancy way of saying that I got a PhD in how nutrition affects our risk of major disease. I also hold Masters Degrees in

Exercise Science and Human Nutrition. I'm a Licensed Nutritionist in the state of Massachusetts, a Certified Nutrition Specialist, and I've been an ACE (American Council on Exercise) Certified Personal Trainer for over 15 years.

I also founded a nutrition counseling and personal training company called Fitness Plus, first in New York, and later in Boston. For the past 15 years, I have helped people lose weight and reduce their risk of chronic disease. I've also spent considerable time in the past few years teaching graduate school, doing corporate and research consulting, and lecturing on health and fitness.

So, what does this book teach you that the first one does not? Well, *The Weight Loss Triad* was a very technical look at each and every element of how to lose weight and keep it off. It not only laid out the steps to successful weight loss, but explained the science behind them. Over the past 15 years, I've fielded a ton of questions on how to incorporate the principles of *The Weight Loss Triad* into the very busy lives of my clients. There were so many questions that there was enough material for a new book. This book is a companion to *The Weight Loss Triad* in every sense of the word. It will help you apply all that you learned in the first book more completely into your life. It will also help you navigate the obstacles to healthy eating that come up for all of us this day and age.

If you haven't read the first book, don't worry. The first section of this book is a brief summary of the program. Of course, this summary will not be as detailed as the first book. However, it will provide you with exactly what you need to be doing with regards to your diet, cardio, resistance training, and lifestyle to get amazing results.

Here's what you'll find in *Life On The Triad:*

Chapter 1: The introduction that you are reading right now!

Chapter 2: A brief synopsis of my first book, *The Weight Loss Triad.* While not as detailed as the first book, this synopsis will summarize the three major components of your weight loss program. The reason I included the summary is that I wanted this book to stand alone. In other words, if you have never read my first book, I want you to find everything you need right here in these pages.

Chapter 3: The 28 Day Meal Plan. This chapter will present 28 breakfasts, lunches, and dinners that strictly conform to the *Triad* principles. You will find meals that are quick to prepare, meals that are highly portable, and a good number of delicious, gourmet selections. The goal of this plan is to provide meal ideas for whatever life throws at you.

Chapter 4: Meal Plan Notes. For those of you who won't follow the meal plan word for word but will pick and choose meals randomly, I included some notes to make sure you remain nutritionally balanced. This chapter also includes sections on portions, snacking, and splurge meals.

Chapter 5: Recipes. In this chapter I provide 28 recipes from the meal plan. These are a step up in terms of quality and taste. Although I'm an OK cook when it comes to the basics, I wanted to bring in the big guns to help with the recipes. I had to look no further than my own family for the help I needed. My sister, Diana Halton, just happens to be an outstanding chef. She graduated from New York City's prestigious Institute of Culinary Education, and I can tell you first hand from our family gatherings that her food is awesome! Her recipes will take a bit more prep time, but man, is it worth it.

Chapter 6: Eating Out. In this chapter, we'll go through some strategies to help you stay in control when eating out at restaurants.

Chapter 7: Travel. Many of my clients are high powered executive types who travel often for work. In this chapter, I'll share some of the successful strategies that we've come up with to help them stay on track during their business trips. We'll also go over some tips to help minimize damage on vacations.

Chapter 8: The Sugar Free Life. In this chapter, I'll teach you everything you wanted to know about the world of sugar free living, including the best sugar free treats and where to get them.

Chapter 9: Shopper's Guide. In this short chapter, I'll list out the foods you should always keep on hand so you'll never be at a loss to prepare a delicious and healthy meal that follows the *Triad's* principles.

There you have it. If you've read *The Weight Loss Triad* and have been following it for some time, this book will give you a bunch of information that will make it work even better for you. If you are new to *The Weight Loss Triad*, then you'll find the answer to all of your weight loss questions in these pages. Are you ready? Are you psyched? Let's get to it.

Chapter #2
Summary Of The Weight Loss Triad Program

As mentioned previously, this chapter will be a brief summary of *The Weight Loss Triad*. I wanted this second book to stand alone. In other words, if you've never read *The Weight Loss Triad*, I still want this book to be complete and work for you. On the other hand, if you have read my first book, a little repetition never hurts, particularly when it comes to healthy lifestyle habits.

The program is called The Weight Loss Triad, and now is a great time to explain just what that means. A triad is simply a group of three. The Weight Loss Triad is comprised of the three areas that you'll need to focus on if you want to lose weight and keep it off for good. More specifically, The Weight Loss Triad is your diet, cardiovascular exercise program, and resistance training. All three of these areas need expert attention if you want to permanently change your body and your life. When people fail at the weight loss game, it is usually because one of these key areas has been ignored or dealt with incorrectly. It is easy to think of these three areas as a pyramid.

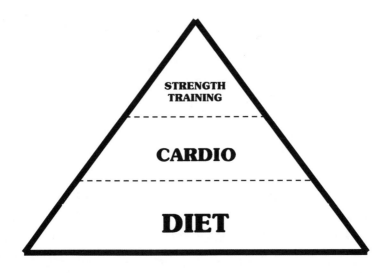

As with any pyramid, the most important part is the base—in this case, your diet. The next most important part is cardiovascular exercise, and last but not least comes resistance training. The pyramid is a quick and simple way to show you how to prioritize the components of this program.

In my experience, for those trying to lose weight, 50% of their results will come from their diet, 30% will come from their cardiovascular exercise, and 20% from resistance training. The pyramid is a rough guide to let you know how you should divide your valuable time and energy.

The goal for the dietary component is to ensure a stable blood sugar. Humans were designed to have a very stable blood sugar, and most of the foods put on this Earth for us to consume promote blood sugar stability. In recent years, we have dramatically changed our food supply by processing and refining foods to the point that they barely resemble the foods we were intended to eat. Getting back to a stable blood sugar will decrease cravings and set your body up for fat burning instead of fat storage.

The goal of the cardiovascular exercise program is, quite simply, to burn calories. This will help to reduce your body fat. The goal of the resistance training program is two fold. As we age, we start to lose muscle. Muscle is a metabolically active tissue, which means that it takes a lot of calories to maintain muscle. The first goal of the weight training component is to not only stop the loss of lean muscle tissue, but to add to it so you burn more calories every day, just by breathing.

The second reason has to do with the human defense mechanism to hold on to body fat. When you lose weight, your body gets nervous and wants to protect its fat stores for the future. Therefore, it will give up a bit of fat, but after a point will start to burn muscle in addition to fat. If you lose weight without resistance exercise, up to 50% of your weight loss is muscle loss. If you add some weight training to the mix, almost all of the weight you lose is fat. This results in permanent weight loss.

So, I hope it's clear that losing weight requires a comprehensive approach. Let's take a look at each of these three components: diet, cardiovascular exercise, and resistance training, in a bit more detail. Again, all of these concepts are very well explained in my first book, *The Weight Loss Triad.* Here we will just summarize the major concepts and then get to the meal plan and recipes.

Diet

As mentioned previously, your diet is the most important component of your weight loss program, and will have the biggest impact on your success or failure. It's time you learned to eat for success! The foods we eat can be broken down into three basic macronutrients: protein, fat, and carbohydrate. Although most foods contain all three of these macronutrients, one is usually represented much more than the others. In this section of the book, I will briefly explain the function of each of these macronutrients, and provide guidance on how to choose the best foods to help you lose weight and improve your health.

The foods put on this Earth for us to consume, for the most part, have a very easy effect on our blood sugar. When we eat these natural foods, our blood sugar rises gradually, and we release a small amount of insulin to lower it back down. This is the way it should be. However, when we eat processed, refined carbohydrates, our blood sugar levels rise sharply, and we need to release a large amount of insulin to handle this peak.

These large swings in blood sugar and insulin have a variety of negative effects for those trying to lose weight. They may actually promote fat storage and inhibit access to fat stores, and most important, they keep you hungry all day long. The key to weight loss is blood sugar stabilization.

There are two strategies to keep your blood sugar stable: 1) *Pick the right carbohydrates*. These are low glycemic load carbohydrates, and they won't spike your blood sugar much at all. 2) *Always combine a source of fat, a source of protein, and a source of carbohydrate at each meal.* Fat and protein slow the entry of carbohydrate into the blood stream. When all three macronutrients are consumed together, blood sugar and insulin levels stabilize. This is the ultimate goal. Now let's go through each of the three macronutrients, and cover the best choices to improve your health and get the weight off for good.

Protein: The Overlooked Macronutrient

Protein is a great macronutrient to start with because most people already know what foods are high in protein, and almost all of these foods are permitted. Eating enough protein is of paramount importance to the maintenance of optimal health. Aside from water, protein forms the major portion of a lean human body, just about 16% of total body weight.

Some of the major functions of protein include:

1) Formation of vital body compounds: like muscle, enzymes, lipoproteins, and hormones.

2) Maintaining acid/base balance.

3) Ensuring fluid balance.

4) Immune function: protein contributes vital parts of the cells used by the immune system.

5) Protein can be used as an energy source for the body.

6) Protein is used to form glucose.

Make sure you include some protein every time you eat! Protein slows the entry of carbohydrate into the blood stream. In this way, it helps promote a stable blood sugar. Protein provides satiety, and can decrease subsequent energy intake. Protein has a higher dietary thermogenesis than fat or carbohydrate, so it burns more calories to process than the other macronutrients.

Your goal should be 20-25% of calories as protein. Limit consumption of proteins that come with a lot of saturated fat and/or cholesterol, as these have a negative impact on risk of heart disease. Limiting red and processed meat is also a good idea. They have both been associated with an increased risk of colon cancer. Here is a list of the *Best Choices, OK Choices,* and *Those to Avoid* for protein.

Best Choices*

Chicken w/o skin	Monkfish
Turkey w/o skin	Flounder
Chilean Sea Bass	Other Fish
Scrod	Egg Whites
Lobster	Black Beans
Crab	Pink Beans
Scallops	Navy Beans
Clams	Chick Peas
Mussels	Lentils
Salmon	Other Beans
Tilapia	Hummus

Can be consumed regularly. These sources of protein are low in saturated fat and should form the core of your protein choices. Shoot for around 3 or 4 servings of seafood per week, but not more than that.

OK Choices*

Skim milk	Filet Mignon
Low-fat Cottage Cheese	Lean Ground Beef
Low-fat Cheese	Lean Roast Beef
Fat Free Plain Yogurt	Pork Tenderloin
Whole eggs	Tuna, Chunk Light
Soy Protein	Shrimp

Can have a few times each week. These choices are pretty good but something about them makes me hesitate to recommend them for every day service. For example: whole eggs and shrimp are high in cholesterol, red meat when cooked may form harmful substances called nitrosamines that may cause cancer, dairy has a variety of problems covered in the next section. Try to shoot for no more than one serving of red meat or pork tenderloin each week.

Strictly Limit*

Whole Milk	Pastrami
Whole Cottage Cheese	Bologna
Whole Yogurt	Sausage
Whole Cheese	Hot Dogs
Hamburger	Bacon
Steak	Pork
Salami	Ham
Pepperoni	Fatty Deli Meats

These are foods that are known to adversely affect your health due to excessive saturated fat or the addition of nitrates or other harmful food additives.

A Note About Dairy

I have serious reservations about the large number of servings of dairy that are recommended by dietitians and other health professionals. No animal consumes milk after the age of six months to a year. No animal consumes another species' milk, ever! So, from an evolutionary standpoint, should we really be drinking a ton of milk? I don't think so. On the other hand, dairy is one of the best sources of calcium in our diet. Calcium plays an important role in bone health. Therefore, I don't advocate completely eliminating it. Five or so servings a week of dairy is what I have my clients shoot for.

A Note About Fish

Fish are an excellent source of protein and omega 3 fatty acids. You may have been reading in the papers about mercury toxicity in our fish supply. This is a legitimate concern, particularly for women who are pregnant or trying to become pregnant. While mercury toxicity can cause a variety of symptoms in humans, it is particularly harmful to developing fetuses. Specifically, it can cause a decreased neurological development.

The larger and more predatory fish tend to accumulate the highest levels of mercury and should be avoided by pregnant women, women who are trying to become pregnant, nursing mothers, and small children. They are swordfish, shark, king mackerel, albacore tuna, and tilefish. I'd go easy on these fish even if you aren't pregnant. If you are pregnant, trying to become pregnant, or nursing, talk to your doctor about the right type and amount of seafood you should be consuming. For the rest of us, feel free to enjoy other sources of seafood three or four times per week, but not much more than that.

Fat: The Misunderstood Macronutrient

Fat is without a doubt the most misunderstood nutrient in the field of nutrition. Fats, also known as lipids, are a wide variety of compounds that share one common trait: they do not dissolve readily in water. Some of the functions of fat include:

1) Providing energy for the body.
2) Storing energy for the body.
3) Insulating and protecting vital organs.
4) Transportation of the fat soluble vitamins (A,D,E,K).

Fat has gotten a *bad reputation!* Early nutrition research showed that certain fats were associated with an increased risk of heart disease and cancer. Another knock on fat is that it is calorie dense, providing 9 calories per gram. For these reasons, the main thrust of nutrition advice in the 80's and 90's was to drastically reduce the amount of fat in our diets. The motivating force behind this advice was to prevent a variety of diseases and to decrease the incidence of obesity.

However, making such a blanket recommendation concerning dietary fat was akin to throwing the baby out with the bath water. Let's start with the weight gain issue. A variety of epidemiological studies show that there is not a strong association between percentage of dietary fat consumed and body weight. In other words, the percentage of fat in your diet has no real influence on your risk of being obese. This is very likely a surprise to most people. I do admit that the amount of fat needs to be monitored in the diet, but in my years of clinical experience and research, I am not at all convinced that a low fat diet is the path to permanent weight loss or greater health.

On to disease risk. I won't argue that certain fats will increase risk of heart disease. What may be surprising is that other fats significantly decrease the risk of heart disease, particularly when substituted for more refined carbohydrates. The association between fat and cancer is also controversial. Recent studies that were more carefully conducted than earlier research have weakened the hypothesis that dietary fat causes cancer.

Let's get this straightened out! There are four types of fat in our diet. Three of these are natural and one is man made. It is imperative that you get to know these really well.

Trans Fat

Trans fat, also known as partially hydrogenated vegetable oil, is a man made fat. It is produced through the commercial hydrogenation of polyunsaturated oils. Hydrogen is bubbled through the oil at a certain pressure in the presence of a nickel catalyst. This gives the oil a certain mouth feel and extends the shelf life of any product that contains it.

Trans fats are slowly working their way out of our diet. This is largely due to the fact that they now must legally appear on food labels. Since they are considered quite unhealthy, few food manufacturers want them in their products now that you can easily see they are being used. However, you can still find them in some baked goods and processed foods. Avoid them as if they will shorten your life, because that is exactly what they have the potential to do. Research has shown that a high trans fat consumption is associated with an increased risk of heart disease, diabetes, and even some cancers.

Saturated Fat

Saturated fats are fats that contain no double bonds. All of the carbons are saturated with hydrogen. They are found mostly in animal products. In general, saturated fats tend to raise LDL cholesterol levels. Research has shown that high levels of saturated fats may increase one's risk of heart disease. Although it is not necessary to completely avoid saturated fat, it is wise to limit intake. Sources of saturated fat include: fatty cuts of steak, butter, full fat dairy products like whole milk, ice cream and cheese, bacon, and other fatty cold cuts.

Monounsaturated Fats

Monounsaturated fats contain one double bond. Therefore, not all of their carbons are saturated with hydrogen. You'll find these fats in olive oil and canola oil, as well as in a variety of nuts and avocados. When monounsaturated fat is substituted for saturated fat, LDL cholesterol drops. This helps reduce risk of heart disease. When monounsaturated fat is substituted for carbohydrate, HDL levels increase. This will also help reduce the risk of heart disease. This is a healthy fat and should be a significant part of your diet.

Polyunsaturated Fats

These fats are highly similar to monounsaturated fats, but instead of having just one double bond, they have two or more. These fats are found in most nuts and plant oils, like corn oil, soybean oil, and safflower oil. Polyunsaturated fats have also been shown to have a beneficial impact on blood cholesterol, and in studies have been associated with a reduction in risk of heart disease. Omega 3 fatty acids found in fish, canola oil, soybean oil, and walnuts are a very special type of polyunsaturated fat that has been shown to reduce the risk of dangerous arrhythmias, and to reduce the risk of sudden death due to heart disease.

I hope it is obvious to you that all fats are *not* created equal. Some are harmful, like saturated fat and trans fat, and others are beneficial, like mono and poly unsaturated fats. We want to limit intake of the former, and focus on the latter. Here's a list to make it easy for you.

Best Choices

Olive Oil	Pistachios
Canola Oil	Macadamia Nuts
Corn Oil	Any Other Nut
Sunflower Oil	Sunflower Seeds
Safflower Oil	Pumpkin Seeds
Soybean Oil	Avocados
Flaxseed Oil	Peanut Butter
Other Vegetable Oils	Almond Butter
Peanuts	Cashew Butter
Almonds	Pistachio Butter
Walnuts	Smart Balance
Cashews	Olivio
Hazel Nuts	Mayonnaise

Avoid*

Whole Milk	Snack Chips
Whole Cheese	Pies
Whole Yogurt	Cakes
Whole Cottage Cheese	Cookies
Ice Cream	Crackers
Butter	Chocolate
Margarine	Hamburger
Palm Oil	Steak
Coconut Oil	Salami
Hot Dogs	Bologna
Sausage	Pepperoni
Bacon	Pastrami
Cream	Any Trans Fat

These are foods that are known to adversely affect your health due to excessively high levels of saturated and/or trans fat.

Carbohydrate: The Most Important Macronutrient

The type of carbohydrate that you put into your body can literally make or break your goal of lasting weight loss. *Pay very close attention to these next few pages!* Let's start from the top. So, what is a carbohydrate? Carbohydrates are composed of carbon, hydrogen, and oxygen in the ratio of 1:2:1. The main function of carbohydrate is to provide energy for the body, and prevent the breakdown of protein.

The type of carbohydrate that human beings have consumed has changed dramatically over the years. While we were still evolving, the majority of carbohydrates that we ate were fruits, vegetables in their whole form, beans, other legumes, and grains that were highly unrefined. As man became more civilized, this all changed, for the worse!

Back before refrigeration and food preservatives, the transport and storage of food was a huge problem. Whole grains contain a small amount of fat that shortens the amount of time that it takes for the grain to spoil. By refining the grain, this fat is removed. Therefore, early attempts to refine grain were initiated by the noblest of intentions: to keep food edible longer, so fewer people would starve. However, this refining process changed the way our body deals with the carbohydrate in a big way.

Biochemistry 101

Let me give you a brief lesson on what happens to your blood sugar when you eat a carbohydrate containing food. After you eat the carb, your blood sugar levels start to rise. Our body works within a narrow frame of blood sugar. You've got a problem if it goes too high, and you've got a problem if it goes too low. For this reason, the body releases insulin to lower your blood sugar. Some carbs cause the release of a large amount of insulin, while others cause a smaller amount of insulin to be released.

When the right type of carbohydrate is consumed, insulin does its job well, and lowers blood glucose to normal levels. When the wrong type of carb is consumed, the large amount of insulin released does its job too well, and blood sugar levels drop below that which the body considers normal. The body quickly recognizes that its blood sugar is low. In order to raise it back up, it makes you hungry. The very thing you'll crave is a quick release carbohydrate, and the cycle starts all over again. Besides making you hungry, insulin tends to promote fat storage as it is an anabolic hormone. This combination of increased hunger and increased fat storage is devastating for those trying to lose weight.

In summary, all carbohydrate foods are not created equal. Some will raise your blood sugar really high, really fast, causing the release of large amounts of insulin. Other carbohydrates have a slower and more gradual affect on your blood sugar, and do not necessitate a large release of insulin. The glycemic load is a measure that can help us pick our carbs to minimize these swings in blood sugar.

The glycemic load of a carbohydrate is the amount of carbohydrate supplied in a serving of that food, multiplied by that food's glycemic index. The glycemic index, in simplest terms, is a measure of how quickly and how severely a carbohydrate food will elevate your blood sugar. The glycemic load measure takes into account both the quality and quantity of a carbohydrate. This is important because both of these factors have a big impact on your blood sugar.

It should not come as a huge surprise that the overwhelming majority of foods with a high glycemic load are man-made, refined carbohydrates. The big offenders are bread, pasta, white rice, and sugar. Most fruits and vegetables have a much lower glycemic load, and will have a milder effect on your blood sugar. This makes sense because fruits, vegetables, and legumes are the carbohydrates that were put on this Earth for us to consume. These foods are what we evolved with, and it is not surprising that our bodies function best when consuming them.

Therefore, when choosing carbohydrates, we want to focus on lower glycemic carbs like fruits, vegetables, legumes, and whole grains such as brown rice and oatmeal. There are just a few exceptions. For fruits, any are permitted with the exception of bananas and grapes. They have less fiber than other fruits and are, therefore, higher glycemic. For vegetables, the only notable exception is white potatoes.

As a side note, consuming a diet with a high glycemic load has been shown to increase your risk of type 2 diabetes, coronary heart disease, certain cancers, and even possibly Alzheimer's disease. So, consuming a low glycemic load diet not only will stabilize your blood sugar and insulin levels, it will also help protect you from chronic disease in the future.

Best Choices

Apples	Green Pepper
Oranges	Red Pepper
Pineapple	Olives
Blueberries	Carrots
Strawberries	Spinach
Raspberries	Lettuce
Melon	Peas
Grapefruit	Lentils
Watermelon	Black Beans
Mango	Pink Beans
Papaya	Chick Peas
Kiwi	Hummus
Sweet Potato	Other Beans
Broccoli	Other Fruits
Cauliflower	Other Vegetables
Tomatoes	Quinoa
Brussels Sprouts	Brown Rice
Onion	Oatmeal (Not
Radishes	Instant)

OK Choices

Corn

Avoid

White Bread	Other Fruit Juice
Wheat Bread	Soda
Tortillas	Cakes
Wraps	Cookies
Pita Bread	Pies
Pasta	Candy
White rice	Donuts
Bananas	Ketchup
Grapes	BBQ Sauce
White potatoes	Steak Sauce
Crackers	Jams
Rice cakes	Jellies
Popcorn	Sweetened Yogurt
Bagels	Raisins
Pretzels	Other Dried Fruit
Potato Chips	Low Fat Salad
Sugar	Dressing
Orange juice	Anything Else
Tomato Juice	With Sugar!!!

Right now you may be saying, "I'll never be able to give up bread and sugar!" Many of my clients feel this way at the beginning of the program, and I will admit that at first it is a challenge to give up these foods. However, when your blood sugar becomes stable, (usually in just two weeks) these cravings will go away entirely. It's hard to believe, but just try to. After two weeks of eating this way, you won't miss the refined carbs.

I've found that cravings for refined carbs are physiological and not psychological. When you are in bad blood sugar, you often crave quick release carbohydrates to counter the dip in blood sugar caused by higher levels of insulin. It is truly a vicious cycle. When you are in a state of "good blood sugar", these cravings disappear.

The first two weeks can be tough because you go through a kind of carbohydrate withdrawal. You may be a little tired or irritable, and you may even get a headache or two. You will also have some serious cravings for the foods you are limiting. These symptoms are not serious, and will go away on their own after two or three weeks. It is a beautiful thing after these two weeks because your hunger will once again dictate your body's energy needs.

Hidden Sugars

Sugar is everywhere! To avoid it, you must become a big time label reader. For example, ketchup, barbecue sauce, steak sauce, and low fat salad dressings are loaded with sugar and need to be avoided. To find out how much sugar is in a product, look at the food label. Under the carbohydrate category there is a listing for sugar. This is the number of grams of sugar in a serving. You want this number to be as close to "0" as possible. Divide this number by 4, and you'll get the number of teaspoons of sugar in a serving. So, if a food has 18 grams of sugar per serving, that equates to 4½ teaspoons. Stay away from this one for sure!

Note that dairy products like milk, plain yogurt, and cottage cheese have a high number under the sugars column, yet don't taste sweet or have any added sugar. This is because lactose is a naturally occurring sugar found in dairy that does not have an adverse effect on blood glucose, it is low glycemic. So with dairy, you'll need to look at the list of ingredients and make sure that no other sugars are added in to the product.

Food manufacturers use lots of different names for sugars. Following is a list of ingredients that can basically be translated to sugar. This is important to know when reading food labels. Rarely will you see the word "sugar" listed as an ingredient.

Also Known As Sugar

Sucrose
Molasses
Concentrated Fruit Juice
Corn Syrup
Corn Sweetener
Brown Sugar
Raw Sugar
Cane Syrup
High Fructose Corn Syrup
Dextrose
Fructose
Levulose
Maple Sugar
Turbinado
Honey
Dextrin
Glucose
Galactose
Maltose
Beet Sugar
Cane Sugar
Agave Nectar
Cane Crystals
Crystalline Fructose
Evaporated Cane Juice
Invert Sugar
Malt Syrup
Syrup

So, there you have it, carbohydrate quality and quantity are pivotal for those attempting to lose weight. In my opinion, the combination of high glycemic load carbohydrates and low fat diets have much to do with the explosion of obesity in recent years. Decreases in physical activity also play a huge role, but we'll get to that a bit later!

Putting It All Together

Ok, so now we have an idea of what foods we should be eating, and what foods we should be avoiding in order to lose weight and improve our health. Now let's put it all together. The most important thing to remember is the following: *Consume one carbohydrate food, one fat food, and one protein food at each meal.*

This is pivotal to the stabilization of blood sugar, which will facilitate weight loss by decreasing cravings, and possibly by increasing access to fat stores. The addition of fat and protein to a carbohydrate food slows the absorption of the carbohydrate into the blood stream, and this greatly decreases the swings in blood sugar and insulin levels so common in the American diet.

For each macronutrient, I listed out all of the best choices. When planning a meal, pick one food from each list. Try to vary them on a day to day basis, but definitely let your tastes guide you. Let's go through a typical day on the plan starting with breakfast. First, pick a breakfast protein from the list of acceptable protein foods—say, some low fat cottage cheese. Now move over to the fat category and select whatever you want—some peanuts for example. Lastly, look at the carbohydrate group and pick a food—an apple will do nicely. We will worry about portions in just a minute. For now, understand that the choice of a food from each category as being a critical part of the dietary regimen.

Breakfast
Protein—Low fat cottage cheese
Fat—Peanuts
Carbohydrate—Apple

Lunch
Protein—Grilled chicken
Fat—Olive oil
Carbohydrate—Salad vegetables (lettuce, tomatoes, etc)

Dinner
Protein—Salmon
Fat—Canola oil
Carbohydrate—Brown rice and broccoli

Now let's move on to lunch. An ideal lunch would be the following: a big salad with lots of vegetables (carbohydrate), some grilled chicken on top (protein), and some olive oil and vinegar dressing (fat). Get the idea? One from each category, any one you want. How about dinner? Let's start with a nice piece of salmon (protein), some brown rice and broccoli (carbohydrate) sautéed in canola oil (fat). That is how it works. Pretty easy, right? It will take a little getting used to, but once you get started, you'll find it is a flexible way to eat filled with a variety of delicious, healthy foods.

I suggest keeping a copy of the "Best Choices", "OK Choices", and "Those To "Avoid" on your refrigerator. This will help you to keep your focus on proper food selection, particularly while you are planning your shopping.

Portions

I never have my clients weigh their food or get too crazy about portion sizes, but a few guidelines are really important. Let's look at each of the macro-nutrients and talk a little bit about portion sizes.

Protein

While at Harvard, a fair amount of my research was focused on low carb diets like Atkins. On a low carb diet, protein is allowed in unlimited quantities, and you are encouraged to eat as much as you want. In randomized trials studying people following a low carb diet, I found it interesting that protein never really exceeded 20-25% of calories. These people were allowed to eat as much protein as they wanted to, and yet they really didn't go overboard. I have also noticed this with my clients.

The reason for this ends up being quite simple. Protein contains nitrogen, which is difficult for the human body to process, and can be quite toxic at high levels. For this reason, the body tends to limit the protein that it will have to process. In other words, you won't overeat protein. So, the take home message here regarding protein portions is to eat protein until you are full. Your body won't let you go higher than 20-25% of calories, which is exactly where I want you to be.

Carbohydrate

The vast majority of carbohydrates on this plan are very low in calories. Fruits and vegetables contain a lot of fiber and water. For this reason, there really are no limits to the amount of fruits, vegetables, and other allowable carbs on this program. Eat until you are full. A big bowl of broccoli will run you about 130 calories, while the same size bowl of pasta can be 600 calories. Load up on a variety of fruits and vegetables without stressing too much about portion sizes.

Fats

Fat is the only one of the macronutrients that needs strict portion guidelines. Having too little fat in your diet will cause you to have blood sugar stabilization issues. Having too much fat in your diet will cause you to have calorie issues. Follow these portions to avoid both scenarios. These portions are per meal.

For Women

1) If you are having oil, mayo, nut butter, or butter substitute: 1 tablespoon will do it.
2) If you are having nuts: 7 large nuts (cashews, macadamia nuts, walnuts, almonds) will do, 14 small nuts, like peanuts or pistachio nuts will do.
3) If you are having seeds: a small handful, just the palm of your hand.
4) If you are having avocado as your fat source: ¼ if it's a large avocado, and ½ if it's a small avocado.

For Men

1) If you are having oil, mayo, nut butter, or butter substitute: 1½ tablespoons will do it.
2) Nuts: 12 large and 24 small.
3) Seeds: a small handful, just the palm of your hand.
4) Avocado: ½ if it's a large avocado, and ¾ if it's a small avocado.

A note concerning beans and eggs

Most foods fit neatly into either the protein, fat, or carbohydrate category. A few foods overlap and really fit into two groups. Eggs, eaten whole with the yolk, provide both protein and fat. Therefore, if you have eggs at a meal, they will satisfy both your protein and fat requirement, and all you'll need is a carb. If you are just using the egg whites, then count them just as your protein. Beans and other legumes similarly are a good source of both protein and carbohydrate, and should be counted as a source in both groups when planning meals.

A Note On Sodium

The impact of sodium on health has been a very hot topic in the nutritional literature of late. Public health efforts to reduce sodium in our foods are becoming more and more focused. In years past, sodium restriction was only recommended for those with hypertension. It is now becoming clear that we all should be limiting our sodium intake. High sodium diets have been associated with hypertension, stroke, heart disease, osteoporosis, and even gastric cancer. A good goal is 1,500 mg of sodium per day. The typical American gets 3,400 mg. Here are a few strategies for reducing sodium in your diet.

1) *Limit processed foods*: This is where Americans get the vast majority of their sodium. Eating food in its natural form is the way to go. Thankfully, the meal plan presented in this book is based almost entirely on whole, natural foods.

2) *Choose low sodium versions of foods when you can*: You can now find low sodium versions of foods all over the supermarket. Choose low sodium soups, turkey breast, turkey bacon, beans, etc. This is an easy way to save hundreds of milligrams of sodium per day.

3) *Don't add any salt at the table*: Better yet, don't even have a salt shaker on the table.

4) *Eat out less*: Always keep in mind that the goal of any chef is to make food taste good, not be healthy. You'll find a lot more salt, sugar, and fat on your plate at a restaurant than at home. If you limit dining out at restaurants, you'll limit your sodium as well.

So this concludes the all important diet component of the plan. Now it is time to focus on the next two areas: cardiovascular training and resistance training.

Cardiovascular Exercise

After your diet, cardio is the second most important factor that will determine your success in losing weight and keeping it off. First of all, cardiovascular exercise burns calories. This will help to access the undesirable fat stores you are looking to reduce. Believe it or not, this isn't even the major benefit of cardiovascular exercise. For about 12 hours after a cardio session, you burn more calories than you would if you had not exercised.

This happens for a variety of reasons, including the reloading of energy substrate and the repair of micro damage to utilized muscle groups. This metabolic boost, in my opinion, is the real benefit to cardiovascular training.

There are three basic components to a cardiovascular exercise program that need to be addressed: 1)Type 2)Frequency/Duration 3)Intensity.

Note

Before we get started, I recommend that you mention to your doctor that you are starting an exercise program, and want to make sure that you are medically cleared to do so. This is very important, and I will not recommend any exercise for a new client until I receive medical clearance. I will be asking you to work at a moderate to high intensity with regards to heart rate, and it's important that you have the confidence that it is safe to do so. Now let's break down the 3 parts of the cardio program.

Type

The type of cardiovascular exercise you engage in is entirely up to you. Let your individual preferences guide you. However, do realize that some exercises are more effective in helping you achieve your goal of lasting weight loss.

Best Choices
Elliptical trainer
Walking or Walk/Jog Intervals
Stair climber

Secondary Choices
Bike
Roller Blading
Ice Skating
Swimming
Jogging
Aerobic dance

Elliptical Trainer

You may have seen these machines on television or at the gym. God bless the man or women that invented the elliptical trainer! This is always my first choice of cardio for my clients, regardless of their age or fitness level. You get the best of both worlds with the elliptical trainer. It provides the calorie burning potential of a more strenuous method of cardio (like running) with very low impact. There is minimal stress on joints with these machines. The movement is very fluid, and a lot of fun. Just about every gym has elliptical trainers, and there are low costing models for the home. The Gazelle Edge is an elliptical trainer that folds up for storage and costs about $100 on amazon.com. I'd say 90% of my weight loss clients have picked one up for their home and love it the way I do.

Walking or Walk/Jog Intervals

If you are 20 to 30 pounds overweight, or are a little bit older (older than 50), you may want to start with brisk walking as your source of cardio. It is an easy, convenient, and cheap way to get started on your cardio. However, after a short while, walking will no longer be intense enough for you to continue losing weight. You'll know this time is upon you when the scale stops moving. At this time, you'll want to graduate to a walk/jog interval training program.

With this type of program, you jog for 2 minutes, and then walk for 3 minutes, and repeat this interval throughout your cardio session. You'll get the benefit of burning more calories than walking, without the continual high impact of running. If the jog/walk interval doesn't sound like your thing and you want to continue walking, count walking for half. For example, if you walk for 40 minutes, count 20 minutes toward your cardio for that day.

Stair Climber

The stair climber is also a great form of cardio that qualifies for the "Best Choice" group. These have been around for years, and do a good job of burning calories while keeping the impact on your joints to a minimum.

Secondary Forms Of Cardio

The secondary forms of cardio are adequate choices, yet are not quite what we are looking for as a consistent choice of cardiovascular exercise. Many of these exercises require a lot of skill, have an increased risk of injury, are weight supported, expensive, or inconvenient. These modes of cardio are fine for a substitute now and again (once or twice a week), but I wouldn't recommend them to be done on a consistent basis. Following is a list of secondary choices and the problems I have with them.

Bike Riding

The bike is supporting your weight, so you are not burning as many calories as you would with a more upright exercise. If you simply love to bike, count 1 minute towards your cardio goal for every 2 minutes you bike. For example, a 40 minute bike ride would count as 20 minutes of cardio.

Roller Blading

This is a great calorie burner but it is not always convenient, and there is a significant risk of injury.

Swimming

The water supports your weight, which tends to decrease the amount of calories burned. Count 1 minute toward your cardio for every 2 that you swim.

Jogging

This is a great calorie burner, but is really tough on your joints. Go easy with this one. I prefer a run/walk over straight running.

Aerobic Dance Classes

Also a great calorie burner, but usually pretty tough on your joints.

Frequency/Duration

The frequency and duration of your cardio simply boils down to a number of minutes you'll need to acquire each week. I have found that it doesn't really matter how you break them up. If you want to workout every day, great. If you want two days off per week, no problem. As long as your minutes add up to your goal each week, the weight will come off. The required number of minutes are specific to men and women.

Women

In my experience, most of my female clients will lose the vast majority of their weight getting 250 minutes of cardio per week. This breaks down to 36 minutes a day if you workout 7 days per week, 42 minutes a day if you workout 6 days a week, or 50 minutes a day if you workout 5 days a week.

Don't jump right into this amount. Work your way up to it. If you are out of shape, start with 120 minutes the first week, then progress to 175 minutes in week two, and then hit 250 minutes by week three.

If you hit a plateau that lasts two weeks or more and your diet has been good, you may want to increase your cardio by 10-20 minutes per week to get the scale moving again. The maximum cardio you should do is around 300-325 minutes per week. If you are getting this amount and not losing weight, cardio is not your problem. Take a close look at your diet and/or lifestyle factors, and most likely the problem will be found there.

Men

Men get off easy when it comes to cardio. Usually 150 minutes is all they will need to lose weight. As with the ladies, if you are out of shape or deconditioned, go easy at first. Start with 75 minutes the first week, then progress to 120 minutes the second week, and then progress to the full 150 minutes by week three.

Similar to the ladies, if you hit a plateau that lasts two weeks or longer, add 10-20 minutes to your cardio to get the scale moving again. In most cases, 150 minutes is all you'll need.

Intensity

The intensity of your cardio program is probably the most important component of the three elements. If you are not working at the proper intensity, the weight loss process will be much less efficient. Generally, you want to workout just below your anaerobic lactate threshold, which is between 70-85% of your maximum heart rate. You may have heard of people taking their heart rate or calculating their target heart rate zone to gauge intensity. Well, I'm not going to ask you to do that. #1) It is complicated. #2) The maximum heart rate formula does not apply to a large segment of the population. #3) There are easier ways.

So, how will you measure your intensity? There are a few simple ways to clue you in to whether or not you are working as hard as you need to be.

1) Are you sweating? After five minutes, you should start to sweat.

2) Can you talk? In the middle of your workout, try talking to someone, even yourself if need be. If you are taking a breath after every two words, you are working too hard and need to slow down. If you are able to string multiple sentences together without

stopping for air, you need to pick it up. You should be able to say a normal length sentence without taking a breath. But you should need to take a breath after this sentence.

3) Ratings of perceived exertion. When you are working out, stop and ask yourself "How hard am I working on a scale from 1 to 10?" If 10 is an all out sprint, you should be at a 7 or 8.

Here are some more tips to help you keep your intensity in the ideal range:

1) When using a machine like the elliptical trainer or stair climber, keep the resistance very low and move quickly. When the resistance is set too high, your leg muscles can tire and prevent you from getting the aerobic minutes you need.

2) When using an elliptical trainer, ignore the arms and just use your legs. I want the focus of the work to be on the large muscle groups of the lower body, and not on the arms. I actually took the arms off of my Gazelle Edge entirely.

3) As your fitness level begins to rise, begin to add some interval training to your cardio. Here's how to do it: Start your cardio at your normal quick pace. After 4½ minutes, increase your speed for 30 seconds. Wear a watch and time this. You don't need to go all out, just increase your speed a bit. After the 30 seconds are over, return to your normal level of cardio for the next 4½ minutes. Repeat these interval sprints 4 times during your cardio session. This is a great way to boost

your calorie burn. I generally reserve interval training for my younger and healthier clients. If a client is very overweight or has risk factors for heart disease (high blood pressure, high cholesterol, insulin resistance), I don't recommend interval training, as the increased intensity can spike heart rate and blood pressure.

Additional Benefits Of Cardio

Imagine if a new medicine was introduced to the market that helped you lose weight. Imagine if this medicine also decreased the risk of heart disease, stroke, diabetes, Alzheimer's disease, and cancer. Imagine if it would also reduce blood pressure, improve your serum cholesterol, increase your energy, and reduce both anxiety and depression. This drug would also combat insomnia, improve your sex drive, and actually increase your confidence and self esteem. Sounds like a dream—too good to be true? This last paragraph pretty much sums up the many benefits of cardiovascular exercise. I know that it is sometimes tough to find the time to fit it in, but you get so much back in return.

Tips For Getting Your Cardio Done

It is not always easy to fit in your cardio. Here are some tips that have helped even my busiest clients hit their weekly cardio goal:

#1) *Make it a priority*—Realize mentally just how important this is for your health and weight loss goals.

#2) *Keep a record of your cardio minutes*—Get a little notebook and jot down your minutes of cardio each day. Accountability makes all the difference.

#3) *Consider getting a piece of cardio equipment for your home*—This has been extremely important for my clients. Very few people can get to the gym every single day. If you exercise outdoors, you've got the weather to deal with, particularly here in Boston! Having equipment in your home means you can always do your cardio. There is no reason to spend a lot of money here. I recommend the Gazelle Edge to my clients. This is a great little $100 elliptical trainer that folds up for storage when you are not using it. I have one myself and love it. Amazon even ships it for free!

#4) *Killing two birds with one stone*—Try to combine your cardio with something you already do every day. Do you read the paper, watch the news, return business or personal phone calls? You can do all of these on your cardio machine, especially if you have one at home.

Resistance Training

Resistance training is the last, but certainly not least component of your weight loss program. It is often ignored entirely by those trying to lose weight. As you will soon learn, this is a huge mistake. Our body can broadly be broken down in two components: fat mass and lean body mass. Fat mass is your body fat. Lean body mass is everything else: your bones, muscles, organs, etc. What you need to realize is that lean body mass burns calories, and fat does not.

Each pound of muscle burns roughly 50 calories each day, even if you don't exercise. These 50 calories are used to maintain the muscle and keep it ready for action. Fat on the other hand, burns next to nothing. As part of the aging process, we start to lose muscle as we enter adulthood. We lose about 1% of our muscle each year after the age of 25. This is a primary reason why people gain weight as they age. Every year, they are burning fewer calories. With resistance training, you can not only prevent this loss of lean tissue, but you can add to it!

It is important to realize that when you lose weight without resistance training, you lose both muscle and body fat. This is the body's defense mechanism to prevent its fat stores from dropping too low, too fast. It is estimated that weight loss without resistance training results in 50% fat loss and 50% muscle loss. This is not good! When you add resistance training to your weight loss program, you lose almost pure fat. This results in permanent weight loss.

Many fear of bulking up and becoming too muscle bound and shy away from weight training, especially women. The type of weight training I advocate is to enhance weight loss and improve health and fitness. You'll notice increased strength and muscle tone for sure, but not large increases in muscle mass. You will be using lighter weights and higher repetitions to help build lean, toned physiques.

Frequency And Sample Program

How many days a week do you need to lift weights? Three is ideal, but you can get away with two. You never want to workout with weights two days in a row. The body needs rest to repair the muscles you use. Therefore, workout on non-consecutive days, such as Monday, Wednesday, and Friday or Tuesday, Thursday, and Saturday. Now I will provide a sample program designed to cover the bases for the weight training component. Each of these exercises will be illustrated in the next few pages. For more information on resistance training, including several gender specific workouts for both men and women, consult my first book, *The Weight Loss Triad.*

Bench Press	3 sets of 10
1-Arm Row	3 sets of 10
Front Raise	3 sets of 10
Bicep Curl	3 sets of 10
1-Handed Overhead Press	3 sets of 10
Squats	3 sets of 10
Abdominal Crunches	3 sets of 10

What Weight Should You Use?

This is a tricky question to address because each person is at a different starting point when I first meet them. Here are some guidelines for men and women, depending on level of experience. Beginners are those who have never lifted weights before. Intermediates are those who have some weight lifting experience, but have not been working out consistently. Advanced are those that have been lifting weights consistently for two years or more.

Dumbbell Weight Guide For Men

Exercise	Beginner	Intermediate	Advanced
Bench Press	8 lbs	15-20 lbs	25-30 lbs
1-Arm Row	8 lbs	15-20 lbs	25-30 lbs
Front Raise	5 lbs	8-10 lbs	12-15 lbs
Bicep Curl	8 lbs	15 lbs	20 lbs
Overhead Press	5 lbs	8 lbs	10-12 lbs
Squats	Chair	Body	15-20 lbs

Dumbbell Weight Guide For Women

Exercise	Beginner	Intermediate	Advanced
Bench Press	5 lbs	8 lbs	10 lbs
1-Arm Row	5 lbs	8 lbs	10 lbs
Front Raise	3 lbs	5 lbs	6-8 lbs
Bicep Curl	5 lbs	8 lbs	10 lbs
Overhead Press	3 lbs	5 lbs	6-8 lbs
Squats	Chair	Body	5 lbs

This is a program designed to enhance weight loss. This program covers the bases for resistance training in the shortest time possible. By all means, if you have the time and interest and prefer a more detailed weight training program, feel free. But for the goal of weight loss and general health, more extensive programs are not really necessary.

Perform the program with 20 second rest periods between each set. Actually wear a watch and time this. I would recommend, if at all possible, that you do your resistance training at home. Invest in a simple bench and some dumbbells. Women can pick up individual sets of dumbbells: 3's, 5's, and 8's are all they will need. Men may want to purchase adjustable, plate loaded dumbbells that go from 5 to 25 or 30 lbs. You may also want to pick up a basic flat bench, but this is not completely necessary as you can do these exercises on the floor with a mat. This equipment won't cost you much, and the routines will typically take only 20-25 minutes to get through. This is probably less time than it takes to drive to and from the gym and change your clothes.

What About Progression?

Start the exercises with 3 sets of 10 reps, and slowly work your way up to 3 sets of 12. When this becomes easy, increase your weights and drop back down to 3 sets of 10 reps. Take your time increasing your reps and weights, this is not a race. Only increase a few repetitions each month.

Your muscles will begin to get used to the challenges that these exercises present, and will eventually stop reacting and growing. For this reason, after 6-8 weeks, it's a good idea to switch up your exercises in order to keep your muscles guessing. In my first book, *The Weight Loss Triad,* I actually provide two different workouts that you can alternate in order to keep your muscles confused.

These exercises are pretty basic. However, if you feel intimidated or unsure, consider hiring a personal trainer for a session or two. I recommend you hire a trainer with a degree in exercise science (Bachelors or preferably a Masters) and at least one nationally recognized certification, such as The American Council On Exercise (ACE) or The American College Of Sports Medicine (ACSM). Remember, although not as important as your diet and cardio, it is essential that you fit at least two and preferably three weight training sessions per week in order to hit your weight loss goals.

Guide To Resistance Training Exercises
Bench Press

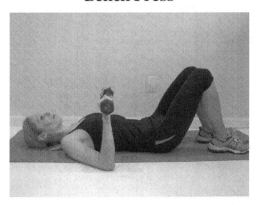

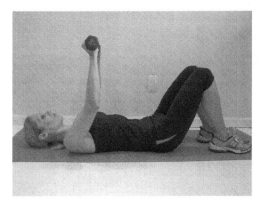

Targets: Chest and Triceps
1) Lie on bench or floor with your back flat and your feet on the floor.
2) Hold dumbbells at the sides of your chest along the line of your sternum (breast plate).
3) Lift dumbbells toward the ceiling.*
4) Slowly return to starting position.

*With this exercise and all others, exhale during the active phase of the exercise, when you are working against gravity. Inhale when you are working with gravity in the passive phase of the exercise. Don't hold your breath! Holding your breath may cause your blood pressure to rise to a dangerous level.

1-Arm Row

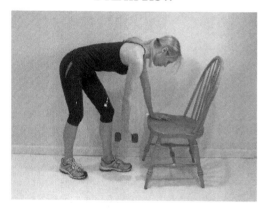

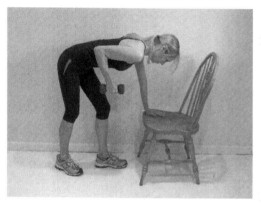

Targets: Back
1) With your left arm on a bench or chair, hold a dumbbell in your right hand.
2) Let your arm hang directly down in front of your shoulder.
3) Slowly pull the dumbbell up toward your chest.
4) Slowly lower the dumbbell to starting position.
5) Keep your back flat and centered over the bench. Your elbow should be tight against your ribcage as you lift and lower the dumbbell.
6) Alternate sets between your right and left hand.

Front Raise

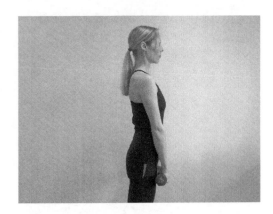

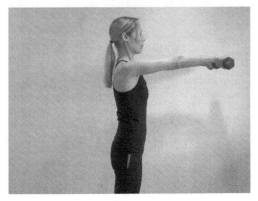

Targets: Shoulders
1) Stand up straight with your feet shoulder width apart.
2) Hold dumbbells directly in front of you with your palms facing your thighs.
3) Slowly raise dumbbells to shoulder level (no higher).
4) Slowly lower to starting position.

Bicep Curl

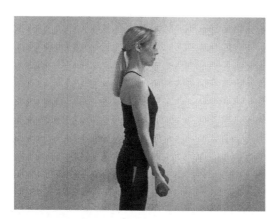

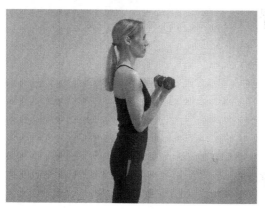

Targets: Biceps
1) Stand with your feet shoulder width apart and your knees slightly bent.
2) Hold dumbbells with your arms at your sides and your palms facing forward.
3) Keep your shoulders still, and slowly bend your elbows to raise dumbbells by just moving your forearms.
4) Slowly return to starting position.

1-Handed Overhead Triceps Press

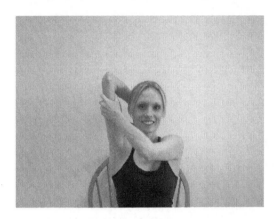

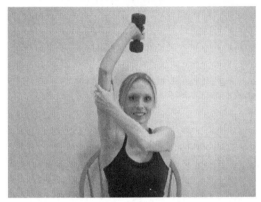

Targets: Triceps
1) Grasp a dumbbell with your right hand behind your head with your elbow bent.
2) Keep your upper arm fixed from shoulder to elbow.
3) Raise the dumbbell toward the ceiling until your arm is straight.
4) Slowly return to starting position.
5) Alternate sets with right and left hand.

Squats

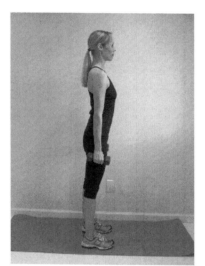 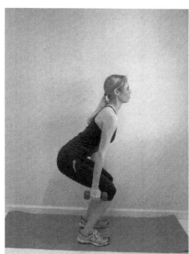

Targets: Legs
1) Stand upright with your feet shoulder width apart.
2) Hold dumbbells at your sides.
3) Bend your knees until your thighs are almost parallel to the ground.
4) Slowly return to starting position.
5) Don't let your knees cross the plane of your toes.

Note: Beginners can do this one by sitting on a chair, placing their hands on their thighs and standing up. Intermediates can do this with their body weight. Advanced exercisers can use dumbbells as shown above.

Abdominal Crunches

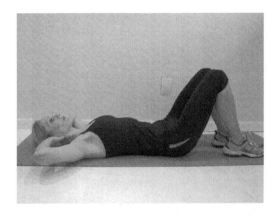

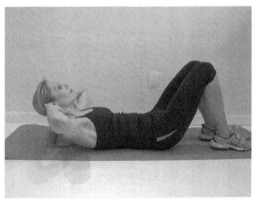

Targets: Stomach (abdominals)
1) Lie on your back with your knees bent and your feet flat on the ground.
2) Put your hands behind your head with your elbows pointing outward.
3) Curl your body upward toward your thighs, until your trunk reaches a 45° angle with the floor.
4) Slowly lower to starting position.
5) Keep your feet on the floor at all times.

Lifestyle Factors

Ok, so we've covered the big three components of the program: diet, cardiovascular exercise, and resistance training. Following are lifestyle and behavioral factors that will go a long way in helping along the weight loss process.

#1 Keep A Record Of Your Diet And Cardio Minutes

I have found that clients who write down their food and cardio minutes are much more likely to succeed in changing their diet and losing weight. Knowing that you have to answer to someone, even if it is yourself, helps you to make better choices. It is accountability! It will also enable you to assess situations in your life that make it difficult to eat well. Appropriate changes can then be made.

I have my clients write down their food for the first couple of months. After that, eating right becomes second nature for them. Here's an example of a typical food log. Just jot down your fat, protein, and carbohydrate for breakfast, lunch, and dinner, and then fill in your cardio minutes for the day. It will take you just two minutes to do, and will truly help you get control of your eating.

Monday July 18th   **Cardio Minutes:** 45 minutes

Breakfast: Protein: Non-fat plain yogurt

          Carbohydrate: Strawberries and blueberries

          Fat: Peanuts

Lunch: Protein: Tuna Fish

          Carbohydrate: Salad vegetables

          Fat: Olive oil based dressing

Dinner: Protein: Chicken breast

          Carbohydrate: Brown rice, vegetable stir-fry

          Fat: Canola oil used in stir fry

#2 No Eating After 8:00 PM

The research goes back and forth on this one. However, there is not a doubt in my mind that if you eat food late at night, the weight won't come off. In fact, now and again I'll get a client looking to gain weight. Having them eat after 8:00 PM is my most successful strategy to get them to pack on some pounds.

#3 Drink 8 Glasses Of Water Each Day

Water increases satiety. Drinking a glass of water or two before a meal can decrease caloric consumption. There is also evidence that our body needs a lot of water to break down fat. If you are dehydrated, the process may be slowed down. Decaf coffee, tea, and naturally flavored club soda (like Polar or Poland Spring) all count toward your water requirement. Try to sip it throughout the day instead of chugging two or three glasses at a time. This is to avoid having to run to the bathroom often, which is the biggest complaint I get on this one.

#4 Limit Alcohol To 4 Drinks Per Week

#1) Alcohol is calorie dense at 7 calories per gram.

#2) There is some evidence that alcohol decreases metabolic rate for several hours after consumption.

#3) After a few drinks, inhibitions go out the window, and the dessert menu or late night diner stop become all but inevitable.

Total elimination of alcohol is not necessary, but I've found that more than 4 drinks per week can slow weight loss significantly, so keep the alcohol to 4 or fewer drinks per week.

#5 Limit Non-Nutritive Sweeteners

The increased prevalence of type 2 diabetes and the popularity of low carb diets have created a gigantic market for sugar free products. It is now common to see sugar free ice cream, cookies, candies, and protein bars, in addition to the all too familiar diet soda. The sweeteners used in these products are fairly well tested and overall pretty safe when used once in a while.

An occasional diet soda or sugar free candy won't do much harm and can be a real treat. However, don't go overboard with this. Non-nutritive sweeteners tend to perpetuate cravings for sweets and refined carbs, and can increase overall hunger. A big reason why this plan works so well is that your hunger greatly decreases after a few weeks, as do your cravings for sugar and refined carbohydrates. If you are hitting the sugar substitutes too often, you'll never get over these cravings.

There is also evidence that due to the cephalic response, your body is tricked into releasing insulin when you consume these sugar free items, because it perceives the sweet taste as sugar. Insulin spikes are what we are trying to avoid. In light of these issues, limit your consumption of sugar free treats and diet Cokes to once or twice a week. You'll find much more info on sugar free living in Chapter 8.

#6 Sleep At Least 7 Hours Each Night

The literature has recently shown that sleep deprivation is associated with weight gain independent of calories and physical activity. That means that even if your diet is great and your exercise is perfect, you'll still gain weight if you don't sleep enough. It appears that sleep deprivation has a negative effect on levels of leptin and ghrelin, two hormones that dictate metabolism and hunger, respectively. Do your best to get 7 hours of sleep each night.

#7 Planned Relapses (AKA Splurge Meals)

No diet needs to be 100% in order to attain your weight loss or overall health goals. Total deprivation is neither realistic, nor necessary. As part of this plan, you are allowed two meals a week to go completely off your diet. I call these splurge meals a planned relapse because you have total control over them. There is no guilt with these splurge meals because you've done nothing wrong.

I recommend planning one mid-week on a Wednesday, and one on a Saturday. This way you'll never go more than three days without eating something fun that you miss. If it's pizza you miss, have that. If it's a cheeseburger, go for it! The only rule I have my clients follow, is to stay away from sugar. If you have sugar even once or twice a week, you'll end up wanting it all the time. Instead, have a sugar free dessert if you want something sweet after a splurge meal. You can find sugar free ice cream, cookies, candy, pudding, and even cupcakes. Be forewarned that these are sometimes made with sugar alcohols that can have a laxative effect in sensitive individuals. Therefore, start with small amounts of these desserts to see how you react. I've found that most people build up a tolerance to this effect over time.

#8 Weigh Yourself Every Week

Weigh yourself on Wednesday every week, first thing in the morning, in your underwear, before eating or drinking anything. Record the number in your food log. When you eat extra salt, alcohol, bread, or pasta, you can retain several pounds of water for a few days, particularly if you have reduced consumption of these food items. That is why you want to weigh yourself on Wednesday. If you are like most of my clients, chances are that you will splurge on the weekends. By Wednesday, you will have been back on track with the diet for a few days, and water retention will no longer be an issue.

To make sure that your weight is accurate, try to limit alcohol and salty foods for two days before your weigh in. Also realize that you are building muscle with this program, which will add small amounts of weight that may slow down your rate of weight loss on the scale. I always tell my clients to go by how their clothes fit rather than by the number on the scale. Never freak out from one bad weigh in, always look at the average weight loss as your indicator of success.

So how fast will you lose the weight? I have my female clients shoot for ¾ of a pound each week, and my male clients shoot for 1 pound a week. You'll likely lose more at first, but you always want the average to be ¾ of a pound per week for the ladies and 1 pound a week for the guys. I know that ¾ of a pound doesn't sound like much, but this adds up to 36 pounds in a year. People who are successful at losing weight and keeping it off, lose it at this rate.

Maintenance

You need to realize that this is not a temporary weight loss diet or exercise plan. These changes need to become a way of life, and while you don't need to be as strict during maintenance, the last thing you want to do is revert back to your old habits that caused you to gain weight in the first place. Having said that, once you have hit your goal weight, you are not going to have to be quite as strict with your diet and cardiovascular exercise program.

Maintenance of weight loss is highly subjective; it will be different for each person. Continue with your weight training at least twice per week in order to maintain and add to your muscle mass. You can generally add another smaller splurge meal and decrease your cardio by about 20-25%. The goal is to keep monitoring your weight. If you gain a pound or two back, add back a bit more cardio and tighten up the diet. By the time my clients hit the point of maintenance, they have a firm grasp on what they have to do to lose weight. It is now totally under their control.

Chapter #3
28 Day Meal Plan

Hopefully, you have now learned the importance of including a source of low glycemic load carbohydrate, healthy fat, and lean protein at every meal. A stable blood sugar is the key to losing weight and keeping it off. Following are 28 days of healthy eating on this plan. You'll find recipes for many of these meals in Chapter 5.

You'll notice that I have not included portions in this meal plan. Portions are actually quite easy to manage, but are different for men and women. Therefore, I thought it would be less confusing to list the foods for now and cover portions in the next chapter, which will answer common questions you may have regarding the meal plan. At this point, I just want you to focus on the combinations of the fat, protein, and carb at each meal. A cross (†) has been placed beside the recipes created by my chef sister, Diana. These are more gourmet and will take a bit longer to prepare but are well worth the effort.

Day 1: Monday

Breakfast
Hard boiled eggs
Grapefruit

The eggs provide the protein and fat. The grapefruit provides the carbohydrate.

Lunch
Grilled chicken garden salad
Olive oil and vinegar dressing
Sliced pineapple

The chicken provides the protein. The olive oil provides the fat. The salad vegetables and pineapple provide the carbohydrate.

Dinner
Shrimp scampi (Recipe on page 134)
Brown rice
Steamed broccoli and red peppers

The shrimp provides the protein. The olive oil and Olivio in the scampi provide the fat. The brown rice and vegetables provide the carbohydrate.

Day 2: Tuesday

Breakfast
Plain non-fat yogurt
Blueberries
Walnuts

The yogurt provides the protein. The blueberries provide the carbohydrate. The walnuts provide the fat.

Lunch
Tuna pouch
Pear
Cashews

The tuna provides the protein. The pear provides the carbohydrate. The cashews provide the fat.

Dinner
Turkey burger, no roll† (Recipe on page 135)
Black bean and corn salad† (Recipe on page 136)
Steamed vegetables

The turkey burger provides the protein. The beans, corn, and vegetables provide the carbohydrate. The oil in the black bean and corn salsa provides the fat.

† Denotes a recipe created by my sister, Diana Halton, a graduate of Manhattan's prestigious *Institute Of Culinary Education.*

Day 3: Wednesday

Breakfast
Oatmeal
Turkey bacon (low sodium and nitrate free)
Melon
Macadamia nuts

The turkey bacon provides the protein. The nuts provide the fat. The melon and oatmeal provide the carbohydrate.

Lunch
Turkey chili† (Recipe on page 122)
Sliced watermelon

The turkey provides the protein. The beans, tomatoes, onion, and watermelon provide the carbohydrate. The olive oil provides the fat.

Dinner
Splurge ☺

Day 4: Thursday

Breakfast
Oatmeal made with low fat milk
Apple
Peanut butter—mix in oatmeal or spread on apple

The milk provides the protein. The peanut butter provides the fat. The apple and oatmeal provide the carbohydrate.

Lunch
Chicken salad with walnuts and apple over salad greens† (Recipe on page 125)

The chicken provides the protein. The mayonnaise and walnuts provide the fat. The apple and lettuce provide the carbohydrate.

Dinner
Grilled filet mignon
Sweet potato with Olivio or Smart Balance
Steamed broccoli and cauliflower

The steak provides the protein. The sweet potato, broccoli, and cauliflower provide the carbohydrate. The butter substitute provides the fat.

Day 5: Friday

Breakfast
Low fat cottage cheese
Pear
Almonds

The low fat cottage cheese provides the protein. The pear provides the carbohydrate. The almonds provide the fat.

Lunch
Garden salad with sliced turkey breast
Olive oil and vinegar
Fresh raspberries

The turkey provides the protein. The salad vegetables and raspberries provide the carbohydrate. The olive oil provides the fat.

Dinner
Healthy chicken tacos (Recipe on page 137)

The chicken provides the protein. The lettuce, tomatoes, onion, beans, and corn taco shell provide the carbohydrate. The olives and corn taco shell provide the fat.

Day 6: Saturday

Breakfast
Vanilla almond butter oatmeal† (Recipe page 116)
Strawberries

*The skim milk provides the protein. The almond butter provides the fat. The oatmeal and the strawberries provide the carbohydrate.

Lunch
Hummus with cut vegetables
Sliced kiwi fruit

*The hummus provides the protein. The olive oil in the hummus provides the fat. The vegetables, kiwi, and hummus provide the carbohydrate.

Dinner
Splurge Meal ☺

Day 7: Sunday

Breakfast
Huevos Rancheros† (Recipe on page 117)
Orange

The eggs provide the protein and fat. The corn tortilla, salsa, and orange provide the carbohydrate.

Lunch
Romaine lettuce and tomato turkey roll ups
(Recipe on page 126)
Peanuts
Sliced papaya

The turkey provides the protein. The lettuce, tomato, and papaya provide the carbohydrate. The peanuts provide the fat.

Dinner
Salmon en papillote† (Recipe page 138)
Brown rice
Steamed vegetables

The salmon provides the protein. The brown rice and vegetables provide the carbohydrate. The olive oil provides the fat.

Day 8: Monday

Breakfast
Plain non-fat yogurt
Sprinkled with healthy granola† (Recipe on page 118)
Sliced fresh cantaloupe

The yogurt provides the protein. The nuts and seeds in the granola provide the fat. The oatmeal in the granola and cantaloupe provides the carbohydrate.

Lunch
Chicken vegetable soup with brown rice
Apple

The chicken provides the protein. The oil in the soup provides the fat. The vegetables and brown rice provide the carbohydrate.

Dinner
Flounder Florentine† (Recipe on page 140)
Brown Rice

The flounder provides the protein. The egg and Olivio provide the fat. The brown rice, spinach, and onions provide the carbohydrate.

Day 9: Tuesday

Breakfast
Oatmeal made with milk and topped with walnuts
Fresh blueberries

The milk provides the protein. The walnuts provide the fat. The oatmeal and blueberries provide the carbohydrate.

Lunch
Tuna pouch
Sweet potato
Almonds
Grapefruit

The tuna pouch provides the protein. The almonds provide the fat. The sweet potato and grapefruit provide the carbohydrate.

Dinner
Healthy chicken enchiladas (Recipe on page 142)

The chicken provides the protein. The olive oil and Olivio provide the fat. The vegetables and whole grain corn tortillas provide the carbohydrate.

Day 10: Wednesday

Breakfast
Scrambled eggs
Fresh raspberries

The eggs provide the protein and fat. The raspberries provide the carbohydrate.

Lunch
Brown rice sushi (Take out)
Pineapple slices

The fish provides the protein. The avocado provides the fat. The brown rice and the pineapple provide the carbohydrate.

Dinner
Splurge ☺

Day 11: Thursday

Breakfast
Oatmeal (made with water and not milk)
Turkey breast (nitrate free and low sodium)
Pistachio nuts
Strawberries

The turkey provides the protein. The pistachio nuts provide the fat. The oatmeal and strawberries provide the carbohydrate.

Lunch
Avocado and shrimp salad with tomato†
(Recipe page 127)
Sliced mango

The shrimp provide the protein. The avocado and olive oil provide the fat. The tomato and mango provide the carbohydrate.

Dinner
Chicken with mushrooms and port wine sauce†
(Recipe on page 144)
Quinoa
Brussels sprouts

The chicken provides the protein. The canola oil provides the fat. The quinoa, mushrooms, and Brussels sprouts provide the carbohydrate.

Day 12: Friday

Breakfast
Low fat cottage cheese
Grapefruit
Cashews

The cottage cheese provides the protein. The cashews pro-vide the fat. The grapefruit provides the carbohydrate.

Lunch
Lentil soup† (Recipe on page 128)
Orange

The lentils provide the protein. The olive oil and Olivio provides the fat. The lentils, vegetables, and orange provide the carbohydrate.

Dinner
Lean ground beef burger with tomato and onion,
(Without the roll)
Black bean and corn salad† (Recipe on page 136)
Sweet potato fries

The burger provides the protein. The oil in the black bean and corn salsa provides the fat. The onions, beans, corn, and sweet potato provide the carbohydrate.

Day 13: Saturday

Breakfast
Oatmeal made with low fat milk
Almond butter
Watermelon

The milk provides the protein. The almond butter provides the fat. The oatmeal and the watermelon provide the carbohydrate.

Lunch
Southwestern grilled chicken salad
(Recipe on page 130)
Becky's dressing, 1½ tablespoons (Recipe on page 130)
Orange

The chicken provides the protein. The salad vegetables and orange provide the carbohydrate. The olive oil provides the fat.

Dinner
Splurge ☺

Day 14: Sunday

Breakfast
Vegetable omelet
Sliced fresh kiwi

The eggs provide the protein and fat. The vegetables and kiwi provide the carbohydrate.

Lunch
Garden salad with sliced turkey breast
Italian dressing
Pear

The turkey provides the protein. The oil in the dressing provides the fat. The salad vegetables and pear provide the carbohydrate.

Dinner
Chicken stir fry
Brown rice

The chicken provides the protein. The olive oil used in the stir fry provides the fat. The brown rice and vegetables provide the carbohydrate.

Day 15: Monday

Breakfast
Fried eggs
Strawberries

*The eggs provide the protein and fat. The strawberries pro-
vide the carbohydrate.*

Lunch
Grilled chicken garden salad
Olive oil and vinegar
Sliced watermelon

*The chicken provides the protein. The olive oil provides the
fat. The salad vegetables and watermelon provide the carbohydrate.*

Dinner
Broiled salmon
Sweet potato with Olivio (or Smart Balance)
Brown rice
Steamed vegetables

*The salmon provides the protein. The butter substitute
provides the fat. The sweet potato, brown rice, and vegetables
provide the carbohydrate.*

Day 16: Tuesday

Breakfast
Low fat cottage cheese
Pistachio nuts
Apple

The cottage cheese provides the protein. The pistachios provide the fat. The apple provides the carbohydrate.

Lunch
Romaine lettuce and tomato turkey roll-ups
(Recipe on page 126)
Almonds
Pear

The turkey provides the protein. The almonds provide the fat. The lettuce, tomato, and pear provide the carbohydrate.

Dinner
Healthy chicken tacos (Recipe on page 137)

The chicken provides the protein. The lettuce, tomatoes, onion, and corn taco shell provide the carbohydrate. The olives and corn taco shell provide the fat.

Day 17: Wednesday

Breakfast
Breakfast tacos† (Recipe on page 119)
Cantaloupe

The eggs, low-fat cheese, and turkey sausage provide the protein. The eggs provide the fat. The soft corn tortillas and salsa provide the carbohydrate.

Lunch
Tuna pouch
Apple
Cashews

The tuna provides the protein. The apple provides the carbohydrate. The cashews provide the fat.

Dinner
Splurge ☺

Day 18: Thursday

Breakfast
Vanilla almond butter oatmeal† (Recipe on page 116)
Blueberries

The skim milk provides the protein. The almond butter provides the fat. The oatmeal and blueberries provide the carbohydrate.

Lunch
Garden salad with sliced turkey breast
Olive oil and vinegar dressing
Orange

The turkey provides the protein. The olive oil provides the fat. The salad vegetables and orange provide the carbohydrate.

Dinner
Lemon herbed brown rice salad with chicken†
(Recipe on page 146)
Peas

The chicken provides the protein. The brown rice, tomatoes, and peas provide the carbohydrate. The olive oil and pine nuts in the salad provide the fat.

Day 19: Friday

Breakfast
Plain non-fat yogurt
Walnuts
Sliced fresh pineapple

The yogurt provides the protein. The walnuts provide the fat. The pineapple provides the carbohydrate.

Lunch
White bean and red onion tuna salad†
(Recipe on page 132)
Sliced fresh kiwi

The beans and tuna provide the protein. The beans, onion, and kiwi provide the carbohydrate. The olive oil provides the fat.

Dinner
Crab cakes with mango salsa† (Recipe on page 148)
Quinoa
Steamed vegetables

The crab provides the protein. The quinoa, mango, and vegetables provide the carbohydrate. The oil and egg provides the fat.

Day 20: Saturday

Breakfast
Oatmeal made with low fat milk and peanut butter
Grapefruit halve

The low fat milk provides the protein. The peanut butter provides the fat. The oatmeal and grapefruit provide the carbohydrate.

Lunch
Turkey chili† (Recipe on page 122)
Peach

The turkey and beans provide the protein. The beans, vegetables, and peach provide the carbohydrate. The olive oil in the chili provides the fat.

Dinner
Splurge ☺

Day 21: Sunday

Breakfast
Poached eggs in Canadian bacon cups†
(Recipe on page 120)
Fresh raspberries

The eggs and Canadian bacon provide the protein. The eggs provide the fat. The raspberries provide the carbohydrate.

Lunch
Chicken pesto salad† (Recipe on page 133)
Sliced mango

The chicken provides the protein. The olive oil and pine nuts provide the fat. The tomatoes, lettuce, and mango provide the carbohydrate.

Dinner
Beef and broccoli† (Recipe on page 151)
Brown rice

The beef provides the protein. The canola oil provides the fat. The brown rice and broccoli provide the carbohydrate.

Day 22: Monday

Breakfast
Low fat mozzarella cheese stick
Peanuts
Apple

The cheese provides the protein. The peanuts provide the fat. The apple provides the carbohydrate.

Lunch
Lentil soup† (Recipe on page 128)
Orange

The lentils provide the protein. The lentils, vegetables, and orange provide the carbohydrate. The olive oil and Olivio provide the fat.

Dinner
Turkey meatloaf† (Recipe on page 153)
Corn on the cob
1 tablespoon Olivio or Smart Balance on corn
Steamed cauliflower

The turkey provides the protein. The corn and cauliflower provide the carbohydrate. The butter substitute provides the fat.

Day 23: Tuesday

Breakfast
Yogurt parfait† (Recipe on page 121)

The yogurt provides the protein. The nuts and seeds provide the fat. The berries and oatmeal provide the carbohydrate.

Lunch
Hummus with cut celery and carrots
Sliced fresh papaya

The hummus provides the fat and protein. The hummus, vegetables, and papaya provide the carbohydrate.

Dinner
Lemon herbed brown rice salad with chicken†
(Recipe on page 146)
Peas

The chicken provides the protein. The brown rice, tomatoes, and peas provide the carbohydrate. The olive oil and pine nuts provide the fat.

Day 24: Wednesday

Breakfast
Oatmeal made with 1% milk
Walnuts
Blueberries

*The milk provides the protein. The walnuts provide the fat.
The oatmeal and blueberries provide the carbohydrate.*

Lunch
Southwestern grilled chicken salad
(Recipe on page 130)
Becky's dressing, 1½ tablespoons (Recipe on page 130)
Nectarine

*The chicken, black beans, egg, and turkey bacon provide the
protein. The salad vegetables, black beans, and nectarine
provide the carbohydrate. The olive oil in the dressing
provides the fat.*

Dinner
Splurge ☺

Day 25: Thursday

Breakfast
Hard boiled eggs
Grapefruit

*The eggs provide the protein and fat. The grapefruit pro-
vides the carbohydrate.*

Lunch
Black beans with red pepper flake and cashews
Watermelon

*The black beans provide the protein. The black beans and
watermelon provide the carbohydrate. The cashews provide
the fat.*

Dinner
Scallop scampi (Recipe on page 134)
Brown rice
Steamed broccoli and red peppers

*The scallops provide the protein. The brown rice and
vegetables provide the carbohydrate. The olive oil and Olivio
provide the fat.*

Day 26: Friday

Breakfast
Oatmeal made with water
Turkey breast (nitrate free and low sodium)
Pistachio nuts
Peach

The turkey provides the protein. The oatmeal and peach provide the carbohydrate. The pistachio nuts provide the fat.

Lunch
Cobb salad
Olive oil and vinegar dressing
Fresh raspberries

The chicken and eggs provide the protein. The salad vegetables and raspberries provide the carbohydrate. The olive oil provides the fat.

Dinner
Pork tenderloin with spicy red pepper sauce†
(Recipe on page 154)
Sweet potato latkas (Recipe on page 156)
Brussels sprouts

The pork provides the protein. The Brussels sprouts and sweet potato provide the carbohydrate. The vegetable oil provides the fat.

Day 27: Saturday

Breakfast
Huevos rancheros† (Recipe on page 117)
Cantaloupe

*The eggs provide the protein and fat. The corn tortilla, salsa, and cantaloupe provide the carbohydrate.

Lunch
Brown rice sushi (Takeout)
Pear

*The fish provides the protein. The avocado provides the fat. The brown rice and pear provide the carbohydrate.

Dinner
Splurge ☺

Day 28: Sunday

Breakfast
Low fat cottage cheese
Cashews
Fresh pineapple

The cottage cheese provides the protein. The cashews provide the fat. The pineapple provides the carbohydrate.

Lunch
Tuna salad
Nectarine

The tuna provides the protein. The mayonnaise provides the fat. The nectarine provides the carbohydrate.

Dinner
Grilled chicken kabobs
Quinoa
Cashews

The chicken provides the protein. The vegetables and quinoa provide the carbohydrate. The cashews provide the fat.

Chapter #4
Notes On Meal Plan

While working with clients over the last 15 years, I've learned a lot about different styles of eating. I've had clients that prepare gourmet recipes for themselves and their family. Others have needed very quick prep times. Some people are on a tight budget, and are looking to limit their food expenditures. There are people that need to eat meals in their car, on a plane, or in two minutes between meetings. Despite these lifestyle differences, all of these people shared one common goal—to get control of their eating and lose weight.

In reality, most of my clients are all of these people at one time or another. Different career, family, and travel situations can change our eating patterns week to week and even day to day. Therefore, my goal when creating this meal plan was to create solutions for all of these circumstances.

It is my sincere hope that you will find a meal option for whatever life throws your way. I've developed meals that can be eaten on the go, meals with very quick prep times, meals on a budget, and also a good number of gourmet recipes for those occasions when you have the time and desire to make your food very special. It may look funny to see a gourmet seafood salad lunch next to a breakfast consisting of a low fat cheese stick, an apple, and nuts. However, both may be appropriate options for you on different days, and under different circumstances.

How To Use This Meal Plan

There are several ways to use this meal plan. If you want to follow it exactly, day by day and meal by meal, your diet will be just about perfect! However, you can also use the meal plan more as a guide, picking meals here and there that suit your tastes and current lifestyle needs.

If you decide to follow the meal plan exactly, all of the thinking has been done for you. If you decide to use the meal plan as more of a guide, keep in mind that the plan has been built around a number of key guidelines that you'll want to follow. These guidelines are in place to reduce your risk of chronic disease, as well as facilitate weight loss.

1) *Aim for 1-2 servings of whole grains each day.* Whole grains have been shown to have a multitude of health benefits, including reducing the risk of heart disease, stroke, type 2 diabetes, and certain cancers. Examples of whole grains are brown rice, oatmeal, quinoa, and whole grain corn tortillas.

2) *Limit egg yolks to 6 per week.* Eggs are a great food. The yolks, although often criticized, actually provide a lot of vitamins, minerals, and other nutrients. In reality, they are very much like a multivitamin pill. Consuming up to 6 or 7 yolks per week has been shown to be safe in the research literature. However, due to their high cholesterol content, you don't want to go overboard with egg yolks, so don't go higher than that. If you have diabetes, it is a good idea to strictly limit egg yolk consumption. Some research has shown an increased risk of heart disease in diabetics who consumed a lot of egg yolks.

3) *Limit dairy to around 5 servings per week.* Dairy has always been a tough one for me as a nutritionist. I'm not a big fan of dairy products. From an evolutionary standpoint, we are the only animal to drink milk after six months, and the only species to drink another species' milk. The protein in milk was designed for a totally different digestive system than ours (cows have four stomachs). I don't think milk is a natural food for us. I've also found that many of my clients are lactose intolerant or have other, less obvious sensitivities to milk. In general, most of my clients will report a benefit when reducing their dairy consumption. I, personally, hardly ever consume dairy products.

On the other hand, milk is one of the best sources of calcium in our diets. Calcium is important for lots of reasons, including ensuring strong bones. Therefore, I like to include some dairy in my clients' diets, but not too much. A good compromise is 4 to 5 servings per week. Try not to go much higher than this.

4) *Limit red meat to 1 serving per week.* I don't think there is a need to completely eliminate red meat. Lean cuts, like filet mignon or 90% lean ground beef, are fine once a week, and provide a good source of iron that is highly absorbable. However, too much red meat has been associated with an increased risk of certain diseases, including heart disease and colon cancer. The relationship with colon cancer is likely due to carcinogenic heterocyclic amines that form during the cooking of red meat. So if you are picking and choosing meals from the plan instead of following it to the letter, try not to include more than one red meat or pork meal per week. Processed red meats like bacon, hot dogs, pepperoni, salami, and other fatty deli meats are particularly harmful. Be sure to strictly limit these foods.

5) *Shoot for seafood 3-4 times per week, but not much more than that.* Seafood is our best source of omega 3 fatty acids. These special polyunsaturated fats have been shown to have a beneficial impact on risk of heart disease, stroke, and even some cancers. However, good sources of marine omega 3's are often good sources of mercury. Mercury is a toxic metal that accumulates in predatory fish and can cause neurological problems in adults, children, and developing fetuses. To keep mer-cury levels low, avoid the biggest sources: tilefish,

swordfish, shark, albacore tuna, and king mackerel. Also, keep total seafood intake to 3-4 times per week. If you are pregnant, trying to become pregnant, or nursing, talk to your doctor about the amount of seafood you should include in your diet.

6) *Shoot for at least 5 servings of fruits and vegetables each day—more is better.* Fruits and vegetables are the healthiest things that you can eat. They are high in vitamins, minerals, fiber, and antioxidants. People who eat a lot of fruits and vegetables have lower risks of heart disease, stroke, obesity, type 2 diabetes, hypertension, and other conditions. Try to have a piece of fruit with breakfast and lunch and vegetables everywhere that you can squeeze them in.

7) *Get a variety of fruits and vegetables.* You've probably noticed that on the meal plan, I have really tried to vary the fruit and vegetable selections. This was no accident. Each fruit and vegetable has its own unique combination of vitamins, minerals, phytochemicals, and antioxidants. To get the whole spectrum, you really want to eat as many varieties as you can. Let your tastes guide you. If a meal calls for a pear and you just can't stand them, it is OK to substitute another fruit. Just try to eat as many different fruits and vegetables as possible.

8) *Eat a serving of nuts just about every day.* Although often criticized for their high fat content, nuts

are an extremely healthy food. They are a good source of poly and monounsaturated fat, protein, fiber, vitamins, and minerals. They are also low glycemic load and therefore very easy on the blood sugar. Nuts have been shown to reduce the risk of heart disease and type 2 diabetes in the research literature. You do need to watch the portions because they are very high in calories. Nut butters are also a great choice.

9) *Include legumes with your meals at least 4 times per week.* Legumes are a great source of protein and low glycemic carbohydrate. They are high in fiber and really good for you. Make sure you include some black beans, kidney beans, pink beans, lentil soup, hummus, or other legumes at least 4 times per week.

Portions

Although I covered portions in the last section of the book, they are important enough to bear repeating. In the meal plan, I have identified each food as a source of fat, protein, or carbohydrate. Here are some simple, yet important guidelines regarding the portions for these macronutrients.

Protein

In general, your body won't let you go too wild with protein portions. Even people on low carbo-hydrate diets, who are permitted to eat unlimited amounts of protein, never get higher than 20-25% of calories. The reason for this is that protein is difficult for our body to process due to its high nitrogen content. Therefore, your body prevents you from eating an amount of protein that it can't handle. The take home message for you is to eat as much protein as you want at a meal. The highest your body will let you go is 20-25% of calories, which is ideal for weight loss.

Carbohydrate

The carbohydrates permitted on this program are extremely high in fiber and water and low in calories. Therefore, you don't need to place a limit on your carbohydrate consumption. Eat your carbs until you are full. If you want multiple sources of carbohydrate at a meal, like vegetables and a sweet potato with dinner, or oatmeal and a piece of fruit for breakfast, go for it.

Fat

Fats are a different story. Too much fat and you'll have calorie issues, too little fat and you'll have blood sugar stability issues. Follow these exact portion guidelines for fats, which are different for men and women. Pick one of these fats and eat the exact amount at each meal.

For Women

1) If you are having vegetable oil, mayonnaise, nut butter, or butter substitute: 1 tablespoon will do it.
2) If you are having nuts: 7 large nuts (cashews, macadamia nuts, walnuts, almonds) will do, 14

small nuts like peanuts or pistachio nuts will do.

3) If you are having seeds: a small handful, just the palm of your hand.

4) If you are having avocado as your fat source: ¼ if it's a large avocado, and ½ if it's a small avocado.

For Men

1) If you are having vegetable oil, mayonnaise, nut butter, or butter substitute: 1½ tablespoons will do it.

2) Nuts: 12 large or 24 small.

3) Seeds: a small handful, just the palm of your hand.

4) Avocado: ½ if it's a large avocado, and ¾ if it's a small avocado.

In summary, when eating a meal off the meal plan, feel free to eat the protein and carbohydrate until you are full, and follow the fat portion guidelines which are gender specific. For example, look at this meal:

Oatmeal made with skim milk
Peanut butter
Apple

Make a good sized bowl of oatmeal with skim milk, and pick out a nice apple. If you are a guy, you can have 1½ tablespoons of peanut butter. If you are a lady, you can have 1 tablespoon of peanut butter.

What About The Portions For The Recipes?

My sister and I created the recipes with the fat portions for women. We figured that men will generally eat a bit more of the meal than women, so they will hit their fat portion because of their larger serving size.

Snacking

You'll notice that there are no snacks on this meal plan. That is because you are not going to snack on this meal plan! 1) *You won't need to snack.* When your blood sugar is stable, you won't be hungry in between meals. It is normal to be quite hungry during the first 2 weeks of the program as your blood sugar stabilizes. You just have to gut this out. 2) *Calories can add up really fast when snacking.* If you eat an additional 75 calories per day beyond what your body needs, this equates to 8 lbs of weight gain in a year and 23 lbs in 3 years! If you find that you are still hungry in between meals after the first two weeks, eat a little more protein at your meals and you should be fine.

Notes On Splurge Meals

You'll notice that twice a week, on Wednesdays and Saturdays, there is no meal listed, you just see the words "Splurge Meal" instead. Splurge meals are a very important part of this program. As mentioned previously, you don't need to be 100% on your diet in order to attain your health and weight loss goals. If you are good 90% of the time, you'll succeed for sure.

That leaves two meals a week to go off your diet. Eat whatever you want on your splurge meals. If you miss pizza, have that. If you want pasta, go for it. It is not realistic or even necessary to completely swear off bread, pasta, or dessert again. The splurge meal allows you to stay on this program forever, because you are still allowed your favorite foods a couple of times a week. Once your blood sugar stabilizes, you won't even have the desire to eat them more than this. Here's a couple of more notes on the splurge meal:

1) *Don't be afraid to eat your favorite foods.* Don't be shy! Bread, pasta, white rice, a burger, Chinese food, they are all fair game. Have whatever you are missing. There is no guilt because you've done nothing wrong.

2) *Stay away from sugar, even on your splurge meals.* For most people, even one or two servings of sugary desserts a week will kick start cravings and throw them off their diet. Instead, go for a sugar free dessert after your splurge meal. You can now find sugar free ice cream, cookies, puddings, and even candy. Later in the book, I'll list some of the better sugar free items out there (see Chapter 8). If you stay away from the sugar completely, you'll have a much easier time hitting your goal weight.

3) *Stay away from trans fat, even on your splurge meals.* Trans fats are extremely damaging to our health, and there is no place for them in a good diet,

even in moderation. Get into the habit of reading food labels, and if you see trans fat listed in the Nutrition Facts Panel, or partially hydrogenated oil listed in the ingredient list, avoid the product.

4) *Feel free to move your splurge meal to another day.* If you'd rather have a lunch splurge on Thursday instead of a dinner splurge on Wednesday, that is your choice. They are yours to plan any way you want, but only two per week.

5) *Separate your splurge meals by at least a day or two.* Don't do them back to back. This way you'll limit your cravings, and never have to go more than a couple of days before your next splurge.

6) *Remember that these are splurge meals and not splurge days!* The rest of the day you eat clean.

7) *Use your splurge meals strategically.* On Monday, look at your upcoming week and figure out the best times to use your splurge meals. If you have a wedding on Saturday night, use one then. If you are going to a restaurant where you know it will be hard to eat clean, use one on that night. Splurges are great for celebrations or occasions when you are not sure what your food options will be.

Meal Reference Lists

As mentioned previously, my goal was to create a meal plan that is highly flexible. I thought it would be a good idea to list out some meals by category for quick reference.

Meals That Can Be Eaten On The Run

Here are a few breakfast and lunch meals that can be eaten on a plane, train, or even in your car.

Breakfast
1) Hard boiled eggs/apple (Day 1)
2) Fat free yogurt/walnuts/blueberries (Day 2)
3) Low fat cottage cheese/almonds/pear (Day 5)
4) Healthy granola/fat free yogurt/melon (Day 8)
5) Sliced turkey breast/pistachio nuts/apple
   (variation of Day 11)
6) Low fat cheese stick/apple/peanuts (Day 22)

Lunch
1) Grilled chicken salad/oil and vinegar/apple (Day 1)
2) Any other salad on Day 4, 5, 13, 14, 15, 18, or 26
3) Tuna pouch/pear/cashews (Day 2)
4) Hummus/cut vegetables/kiwi (Day 6)
5) Lettuce turkey wraps/peanuts/papaya (Day 7)
6) Brown rice sushi/pineapple (Day 10)

Meals With Really Quick Prep Times

Here are a few breakfast, lunch, and dinner meals that can be put together fast, when your schedule is tight.

Breakfast
1) Plain nonfat yogurt/blueberries/walnuts (Day 2)
2) Oatmeal/milk/peanut butter/apple (Day 4)
3) Low fat cottage cheese/pear/almonds (Day 5)
4) Scrambled eggs/raspberries (Day 10)
5) Fried eggs/strawberries (Day 15)
6) Low fat cheese stick/apple/peanuts (Day 22)

Lunch
1) Tuna pouch/cashews/pear (Day 2)
2) Sliced turkey breast garden salad/oil and vinegar/ raspberries (Day 5)
3) Hummus/cut vegetables/kiwi (Day 6)
4) Lettuce turkey wraps/peanuts/papaya (Day 7)
5) White bean and red onion tuna salad/kiwi (Day 19)
6) Black beans/cashews/watermelon (Day 25)

Dinner
1) Turkey burger/black bean and corn salad/steamed vegetables (Day 2)
2) Filet mignon/sweet potato/broccoli and cauliflower (Day 4)
3) Chicken tacos (Day 5)
4) Chicken enchiladas (Day 9)
5) Grilled chicken kabobs/quinoa/cashews (Day 28)

Gourmet Meals

These take a little more time to prepare but are well worth it! These recipes are designed by my sister Diana, who is a recent graduate of Manhattan's prestigious *Institute of Culinary Education.*

Breakfast
1) Vanilla almond butter oatmeal/strawberries (Day 6)
2) Huevos rancheros/orange (Day 7)
3) Breakfast tacos/cantaloupe (Day 17)
4) Poached eggs in Canadian bacon cups/raspberries (Day 21)
5) Yogurt parfait (Day 23)

Lunch
1) Turkey chili/watermelon (Day 3)
2) Chicken salad with walnuts and apples over salad greens (Day 4)
3) Avocado shrimp salad and tomato/mango (Day 11)
4) Lentil soup/orange (Day 12)
5) White bean and red onion tuna salad/kiwi (Day 19)
6) Chicken pesto salad/mango (Day 21)

Dinner
1) Salmon en papillote/brown rice/steamed vegetables (Day 7)
2) Flounder Florentine/brown rice (Day 8)
3) Chicken with mushrooms and port wine sauce/ quinoa/Brussels sprouts (Day 11)

4) Crab cakes/quinoa/steamed vegetables (Day 19)
5) Pork tenderloin with spicy red pepper sauce/sweet
potato latkas/Brussels sprouts (Day 26)

Chapter #5
Recipes

In this chapter you'll find all of the recipes from the 28 day meal plan. They are listed in order of appearance in the meal plan and divided into *Breakfast, Lunch,* and *Dinner* sections. Some of the recipes are really simple, some are a bit more on the gourmet side. Hopefully, you'll find great options whatever your cooking skills or time for prep may be. You can be confident that these meals will taste great, improve your health, and help you attain your weight goals.

My little sister gets the credit for the majority of these recipes. She is an amazing chef, educated at the prestigious *Institute For Culinary Education* in New York City. My family has been enjoying her delicious concoctions for years now, and I'm glad to share some of our favorites with you. Whenever you see a cross after a recipe name (†), you'll know that the recipe was created by my sister, Diana Halton. These recipes will take a bit more prep time and be a bit more fancy—but trust me, they are well worth the effort!

Breakfast

Vanilla Almond Butter Oatmeal†
Serves 1

What You'll Need
½ cup old fashioned oats
1 tablespoon almond butter
1 cup skim milk
1 teaspoon vanilla extract
½ teaspoon ground cinnamon

Meal Prep
1) In a small saucepan, over medium high heat, add the oats, milk, vanilla, and cinnamon and bring to a boil.

2) Reduce heat and cook until oats reach desired consistency, about 5 minutes.

3) Remove from heat, add the almond butter to saucepan, stir and serve hot.

Huevos Rancheros†
Serves 1

What You'll Need
2 eggs cooked over easy
2 whole grain corn tortillas
2 tablespoons salsa
¼ cup black beans
⅛ avocado
2 tablespoons non-fat sour cream

Meal Prep
1) In a sauté pan over medium heat, warm corn tortillas one at a time until slightly brown on both sides.

2) Crack eggs one at a time into a non-stick sauté pan over medium high heat. Cover and cook eggs until whites are cooked and yolks are runny.

3) Place eggs over corn tortillas. Top with black beans, salsa, avocado, and sour cream.

Healthy Granola†
Serving Size: ½ Cup
Number Of Servings: 8

What You'll Need
3 cups old fashioned oatmeal (not instant)
2 tablespoons flax seed powder
¼ cup unsweetened coconut
¼ cup sliced almonds
¼ cup walnuts
¼ cup sunflower seeds
1 tablespoon cinnamon
1 tablespoon vanilla
3 tablespoons vegetable oil

Meal Prep
1) In a mixing bowl combine oatmeal, flax seed powder, coconut, almonds, walnuts, and sunflower seeds.

2) Sprinkle with cinnamon, vanilla, and vegetable oil.

3) Stir until coated.

4) Spread out on baking sheet, and bake in a preheated 350° oven for 20 minutes, stirring occasionally.

5) Let cool and store in air tight container.

Breakfast Tacos†
Serves 1

What You'll Need
1 low fat turkey breakfast sausage
2 eggs
2 corn tortillas
Salsa to taste
¼ cup fat free shredded cheddar or American cheese

Meal Prep
1) Break up and cook turkey sausage in a sauté pan over medium heat.

2) Beat eggs in a bowl and cook in a separate sauté pan over medium heat until scrambled and fluffy.

3) Gently warm tortillas in a frying pan over low heat for about 30 seconds on each side.

4) Combine egg and sausage mixture and place in center of corn tortillas. Top with salsa and cheese.

5) Microwave for 10-15 seconds to melt cheese.

Poached Eggs In Canadian Bacon Cups†
Serves 1

What You'll Need
2 slices Canadian bacon
2 eggs
Salt and pepper to taste
Sliced melon, 2-3 pieces

Meal Prep
1) Preheat oven to 350°.

2) Place the Canadian bacon into two of the cups of a non-stick muffin baking tin, forming a cup.

3) Next crack the eggs one at a time into a separate bowl keeping the yolks in tact. Check to make sure there are no shells, and then pour one egg into each Canadian bacon cup. Sprinkle with salt and pepper.

4) Bake for 15-20 minutes or until egg is cooked to preferred consistency.

5) Gently remove from muffin tin and serve with sliced melon.

Yogurt Parfait†
Serves 1

What You'll Need
1 cup nonfat Greek yogurt
½ teaspoon vanilla extract
½ cup Healthy Granola (recipe on page 118)
1 cup mixed berries (blueberries, raspberries,
 strawberries)

Meal Prep
1) Mix vanilla and yogurt.

2) Place half of the berries into a parfait or glass cup.

3) Add half of the granola, followed by half of the yogurt.

4) Repeat and serve.

Lunch

Turkey Chili†
Makes 10 servings

What You'll Need
1 bag pinto beans
1 medium onion, quartered
2 cloves whole garlic, peeled

2 teaspoons extra virgin olive oil
1½ pounds spicy turkey sausage, removed from casing
1 pound ground turkey breast
1 large yellow onion, medium diced
1 large green pepper, medium diced
2 cloves of garlic, minced
1 cup red wine
⅓ cup Worcestershire sauce
1 teaspoon dry mustard
1 teaspoon celery seed
1½ teaspoons chili powder
Salt and pepper to taste
2 cans Italian tomatoes, chopped but not drained

Meal Prep

1) Place pinto beans in a medium sized pot and cover with water. Add quartered onion and garlic cloves.

2) Simmer over medium heat for 1-2 hours until beans are tender. Add water as necessary to prevent beans from drying out.

3) In a large pot, heat olive oil over medium high heat and cook turkey sausage, breaking it up while it browns, for 5-7 minutes. Remove and set turkey sausage aside.

4) Add ground turkey breast to pan and cook until browned, approximately 10 minutes. Remove ground meat and set aside.

5) Sauté onion and peppers for 3-5 minutes. Add minced garlic and cook for an additional 2 minutes.

6) Stir in wine and Worcestershire sauce, and let simmer for 10 minutes.

7) Next stir in dried mustard, celery seed, chili powder, salt, and pepper, and simmer another 10 minutes.

8) Chop up tomatoes with juice and add to pot.

9) Simmer uncovered for 30 minutes.

10) Finally add meat and strained pinto beans to pot. Bring to boil, reduce heat and simmer covered, for 1 hour.

11) Chili is best if made the day before serving. Serve with chopped onion, low fat shredded cheddar cheese, and fat free sour cream.

Chicken Salad With Walnuts And Apple†
Serves 2

What You'll Need
½ pound roasted chicken, skin removed, cut into ½ inch cubes
½ cup apple, peeled, cored, and medium diced
¼ cup celery, small diced
2 tablespoons red onion, small diced
¼ cup walnuts, roughly chopped
1 tablespoon low fat mayonnaise
Salt and pepper to taste

Meal Prep
1) In a bowl combine chicken, apple, celery, red onion, and walnuts.

2) Gently mix in mayonnaise, add salt and pepper to taste.

3) Serve over a bed of greens.

Romaine Lettuce And Tomato Turkey Roll- Ups

Serves 1

What You'll Need
Deli sliced turkey breast
Tomato, sliced
Romaine lettuce

Meal Prep
1) Pull off several large leaves of romaine lettuce at the stem.

2) Lay lettuce out flat and place several slices of turkey breast and sliced tomato on lettuce.

3) Wrap lettuce up and cover in foil for a delicious and simple lunch that is highly portable.

Avocado And Shrimp Salad With Tomato†
Serves 1

What You'll Need
5 cooked shrimp, tails removed
¼ avocado, peeled, pitted, and medium diced
1 small tomato, medium diced
¼ cup onion, medium diced
1 tablespoon cilantro, chopped
1 tablespoon lime juice
½ tablespoon olive oil
Salt and pepper to taste

Meal Prep
1) Cut shrimp into 2-3 pieces and place in a bowl.

2) Add avocado, tomato, onion, cilantro, lime juice, olive oil, salt, and pepper.

3) Gently mix and let marinate 30 minutes in refrigerator before serving.

Lentil Soup†
Serves 8

What You'll Need
1 pound dried lentils, picked through and washed
1 large onion, small diced
1 garlic clove, minced
5 carrots, peeled and medium diced
4 celery stalks, no leaves, medium diced
1 (8 oz) can of tomato sauce
3½ tablespoons extra virgin olive oil
2 tablespoons Olivio or Smart Balance
2 beef bouillon cubes
3 quarts water
Salt and pepper to taste

Meal Prep
1) Place lentils in cold water and parboil for 5 to 6 minutes.

2) In another pot, heat the 3 quarts of water and bring to a boil.

3) Using a 4 quart pot for the soup, sauté onion in olive oil and Olivio over medium heat.

4) Add garlic, salt and pepper and cook until onion is soft.

5) Add tomato sauce.

6) Drain lentils and add to mixture.

7) Add the 3 quarts of boiling water and stir.

8) Cover and simmer for an hour.

9) Add carrots and celery, and continue simmering at low heat for another hour, stirring occasionally.

10) If desired, add 2 beef bouillon cubes to soup.

Southwestern Grilled Chicken Salad
Serves 1

What You'll Need
For The Salad
1 (4 oz) chicken breast
2 cups romaine lettuce
¼ cup black beans
¼ cup corn
½ hard boiled egg, sliced
6 grape tomatoes
½ slice turkey bacon, cooked and crumbled
3 olives, sliced
½ carrot sliced
1½ tablespoons Becky's Dressing

Becky's Dressing
1 cup extra virgin olive oil
2 lemons
2 teaspoons minced garlic
½ teaspoon salt
½ teaspoon pepper

Meal Prep
For The Salad
1) Lay out romaine lettuce in a large salad bowl.

2) Grill and slice the chicken breast. We use the George Foreman Grill which cooks the chicken in about 6 minutes.

3) Add beans, corn, egg, turkey bacon, tomato, carrot, olives, and sliced chicken breast.

4) Add 1½ tablespoons of dressing.

For The Dressing
1) Juice lemons and combine with oil, garlic, salt, and pepper in salad dressing bottle. Mix vigorously and serve.

White Bean And Red Onion Tuna Salad†
Serves 2

What You'll Need
1 can cannellini beans, rinsed and drained
1 can solid white albacore tuna packed in water,
     drained well
¼ cup red onion, thinly sliced
2 tablespoons extra virgin olive oil
2 tablespoons balsamic vinegar
Pepper to taste

Meal Prep
1) Place cannellini beans in a bowl.

2) Break up tuna with a fork in a separate bowl and add to beans.

3) Add onions, balsamic vinegar, olive oil, and pepper and gently toss.

Chicken Pesto Salad†
Serves 2

What You'll Need
1 cup grilled chicken breast, chopped into ½ inch cubes
1½ tablespoons pine nuts
½ cup cherry tomatoes, cut in half
2 cups lettuce greens

For The Pesto
2 cups loosely packed basil
¼ cup reduced fat parmesan cheese
1 clove garlic
2 teaspoons extra virgin olive oil
Salt and pepper to taste

Meal Prep
1) Combine basil, parmesan, garlic, salt, and pepper in a food processor.

2) Slowly stream in olive oil while mixing. Stop to scrape down mixture with a rubber spatula. Mix until well blended.

3) In a bowl, lightly toss chicken, pine nuts, and tomatoes with pesto mixture.

4) Place over lettuce greens and serve.

Dinner

Shrimp Scampi (Or Scallop Scampi)
Serves 2

What You'll Need
20 medium shrimp (or scallops), with shells and tails
      removed
3 tablespoons Olivio Light or Smart Balance Light
1 tablespoon olive oil
2 teaspoons minced garlic
1 teaspoon crushed red pepper flakes

Meal Prep
1) Place shrimp in a medium casserole pan. Make sure they are not touching each other.

2) Add Olivio, olive oil, minced garlic, and red pepper flakes.

3) Broil for about 8 minutes, flipping shrimp and stirring sauce at 4 minutes. Cooking time may vary depending on your oven, so keep an eye on them to make sure they are not too crispy.

4) Serve with brown rice and steamed broccoli and red peppers.

Turkey Burgers†
Serves 2

What You'll Need
½ pound lean ground turkey breast
¼ cup onion, small dice
1 teaspoon extra virgin olive oil
1 clove garlic, minced
2 large white mushrooms, small dice
1 tablespoon parsley, finely chopped
1 tablespoon Dijon mustard
1 teaspoon Worcestershire sauce
Salt and pepper to taste

Meal Prep
1) Sauté onion in olive oil, until translucent, for about 3 minutes. Add garlic and mushrooms, and sauté for an additional 3 minutes. Set aside to cool.

2) In a bowl, combine ground turkey, onion and mushroom mixture, Dijon mustard, Worcestershire sauce, salt, and pepper.

3) Mix well, then add in parsley and form into 2 patties.

4) Spray a nonstick cooking pan with Pam. Cook patties over medium heat until they are no longer pink in the middle, approximately 5 minutes on each side.

Black Bean And Corn Salad†
Makes about 7 servings

What You'll Need
1 can black beans, rinsed and drained
1 can corn
½ cup onion, small dice
1 cup red pepper, small dice
2 tablespoons parsley, chopped
½ lemon, juiced
2 tablespoons white wine vinegar
2 tablespoons olive oil
Salt and pepper to taste

Meal Prep
1) Combine all ingredients in a bowl.

2) Set aside for at least 30 minutes and serve.

Healthy Chicken Tacos
Makes 2 servings of 3 tacos

What You'll Need
2 medium chicken breasts
1 cup of romaine lettuce, chopped
¼ cup onion, chopped
1 medium tomato, chopped
¼ cup black olives, chopped
¼ packet taco seasoning, low sodium
6 whole grain corn taco shells
¼ cup salsa

Meal Prep
1) Pre-heat oven to warm taco shells according to directions on package, they usually take about 10 minutes to heat up.

2) Grill and slice chicken breast, place in skillet over low heat.

3) Add 2 tablespoons of water and taco seasoning, mix until all chicken is covered.

4) Place chicken mixture in bottom of warmed taco shells. Top with lettuce, tomato, onion, olives, and salsa.

Salmon En Papillote†
Serves 2

What You'll Need
2 wild salmon fillets, skin on, any bones removed
1 medium red bell pepper, thinly sliced
1 carrot, thinly sliced
1 leek, sliced and rinsed thoroughly (white and light
    green portion only)
1 large clove garlic
2 tablespoons olive oil
¼ cup white wine
Salt and pepper to taste

Meal Prep
1) Preheat oven to 350°. Lay a 12 inch x 12 inch piece of foil or parchment paper down on a baking sheet.

2) Place a seasoned filet of salmon, skin side down in center. Pour one tablespoon of olive oil over salmon, coating thoroughly.

3) Place half of the sliced vegetables on top of the salmon, half of the garlic, and finish with half of the wine.

4) Fold both sides of foil up over salmon and seal edges forming a packet. Repeat with second piece of salmon.

5) Place both packets on sheet and bake for 30 minutes. Serve with brown rice.

Flounder Florentine†
Serves 2

What You'll Need
2 medium flounder fillets
½ pound spinach, chopped, fresh or frozen
½ cup onion, small diced
1 egg, lightly beaten
¼ cup low fat sour cream
2 tablespoons low fat parmesan cheese, grated
1½ tablespoon Olivio or Smart Balance, melted
1 teaspoon lemon juice
¼ cup white wine
Salt and pepper to taste

Meal Prep
1) Sauté onion in 1 tablespoon of Olivio until soft, about 5 minutes.

2) Add chopped spinach and cook for another 3 minutes. Take off heat, set aside in a bowl, and let cool.

3) Once cool, add egg, sour cream, parmesan cheese, and lemon juice to spinach/onion mixture.

4) Slightly flatten flounder fillets between wax paper. Season fillets with salt and pepper. Spread spinach mixture over top of each fillet.

5) Spray baking dish with non stick cooking spray. Roll each fillet and place seam side down on baking dish. Brush fish with remaining Olivio and sprinkle with white wine.

6) Cover with foil and refrigerate for at least a half hour. Set oven to 425°. Bake, covered with foil for 8-10 minutes. Uncover and broil for an additional 2-4 minutes, until browned.

Healthy Chicken Enchiladas
Serves 2

What You'll Need
2 medium sized chicken breasts
¼ cup black beans
¼ cup corn
¼ cup onion, chopped
¼ cup green pepper, chopped
1 tablespoon olive oil
1 tablespoon Olivio or Smart Balance
¼ cup salsa
8 whole grain corn tortillas
1 medium tomato, chopped
2 tablespoons low sodium taco seasoning

Meal Prep
1) Grill chicken breast and cut into bite sized pieces. A George Foreman Grill is ideal for this task, and it will take about 6 minutes for the chicken to cook.

2) While chicken is grilling, add beans, corn, onion, green pepper, Olivio, and olive oil to a frying pan and sauté over medium heat until vegetables are soft.

3) Warm corn tortillas by covering both sides with a damp paper towel and microwaving on a plate for 45 seconds.

4) Add grilled, cut chicken to frying pan with other ingredients. Add taco seasoning and cook while stirring for 2-3 minutes.

5) Fill corn tortillas with a few spoonfuls of the mixture, roll and place on a plate. Cover the tortillas with salsa and chopped tomatoes. Microwave plate for about 45 seconds to warm the salsa, if desired.

Chicken With Mushrooms And Port Wine Sauce†

Serves 2

What You'll Need
4 thin chicken cutlets
Salt and pepper to taste
¼ cup whole wheat flour, for dredging
2 tablespoons canola oil
¼ cup yellow onion, medium dice
1 clove garlic, minced
1 cup Cremini mushrooms, sliced
¼ cup chicken stock
3 tablespoons port wine
1 teaspoon parsley, finely chopped

Meal Prep
1) Season chicken cutlets with salt and pepper. Lightly dredge chicken in flour, shaking off any excess.

2) In a medium sized sauté pan, add canola oil over medium high heat until hot, but not smoking. Add chicken cutlets and cook until golden brown, approximately 3 minutes on each side. Remove cutlets and cover in foil.

3) In same sauté pan, add onion and cook until translucent. Add garlic and mushrooms. Cook mushrooms until tender.

4) Deglaze pan with port wine. Add chicken stock and cook over medium high heat until reduced by half. Serve sauce over chicken cutlets and garnish with chopped parsley.

Lemon Herbed Brown Rice Salad With Grilled Chicken†

Serves 4

What You'll Need
1 cup brown rice
2 cups cherry tomatoes, cut in half
1 tablespoon fresh basil, chopped
1 tablespoon fresh mint, chopped
2 tablespoons pine nuts, toasted
1 teaspoon lemon zest
½ lemon juice
3 tablespoons extra virgin olive oil
Salt and pepper to taste
4 grilled chicken breasts

Meal Prep
1) Cook brown rice according to package directions. Fluff rice and set aside to cool completely.

2) Lightly toast pine nuts in a sauté pan over low heat, watching carefully not to burn them.

3) Combine olive oil and lemon juice in a small bowl, mixing well.

4) In a larger bowl, combine rice, tomatoes, basil, parsley, mint, pine nuts, lemon zest, and olive/lemon dressing. Season with salt and pepper and mix well.

Serve grilled chicken on side or on top of brown rice salad.

Crab Cakes With Mango Salsa†
Yields 4 large crab cakes- 2 servings

What You'll Need
1 pound lump crabmeat, cleaned to remove any shells
  (squeeze crabmeat dry if there is excess moisture)
½ tablespoon extra virgin olive oil
½ cup red pepper, small dice
½ cup scallions, thinly sliced
1 large clove garlic, minced
1 large egg
1 tablespoon cilantro, minced
1 teaspoon old bay seasoning
1 tablespoon Worcestershire sauce
Salt and pepper to taste
¼ cup whole wheat bread crumbs for dredging
Canola oil as needed

Meal Prep
1) Over medium heat, sauté red pepper in extra virgin olive oil for 3-5 minutes. Add in scallions and lastly garlic. Sauté for an additional 2 minutes. Set aside to cool.

2) Mix crabmeat, egg, cilantro, old bay seasoning, Worcestershire sauce, salt, pepper, and red pepper mixture in a large bowl.

3) Form into four equal patties. Lightly dredge patties in breadcrumbs. Place in refrigerator for a minimum of one hour.

4) Coat a non-stick sauté pan with a thin layer of canola oil. Over medium-high heat, pan fry the crab cakes for approximately 4-5 minutes on each side. Remove excess oil by placing crab cakes on plate covered with paper towels. Serve over a bed of greens with mango salsa (recipe on next page).

Mango Salsa[†]
For Crab Cakes

What You'll Need
1 mango, small dice
2 tomatoes, small dice
1 jalapeno, small dice
½ cup red onion, small dice
2 tablespoons lime juice
½ tablespoon olive oil
Salt and pepper to taste

Meal Prep
1) Combine ingredients in a bowl and set aside to marinate for at least one hour.

Beef And Broccoli†
Serves 2

What You'll Need
1½ tablespoons cornstarch
Salt and pepper to taste
½ pound sirloin beef tips, thinly sliced against the
    grain
2 tablespoons canola oil
2 cups broccoli florets, cut into small pieces
2 large cloves minced garlic
3 tablespoons low sodium soy sauce
1 teaspoon fresh ginger root, grated
⅓ cup water

Meal Prep
1) In a medium sized bowl, toss cornstarch, salt, pepper and beef until meat is thoroughly coated.

2) Heat 1 tablespoon of canola oil in a wok or large sauté pan until hot but not smoking. Add beef and cook, stirring constantly for 2-3 minutes. Transfer meat to another bowl and cover with foil.

3) Add remaining tablespoon of canola oil to wok or sauté pan. Add broccoli and cook over medium high heat until just tender. Add garlic and ginger, and cook for an additional 2 minutes.

4) Add soy sauce and water to broccoli and bring to a boil. Return meat to pan, and cook until sauce is thickened. Serve over brown rice.

Turkey Meatloaf†
Makes about 4 servings

What You'll Need
1 cup yellow onion, medium diced
1 tablespoon extra virgin olive oil
1 large clove minced garlic
1 pound ground turkey breast
1 tablespoon parsley, finely chopped
1 teaspoon tomato paste
½ cup whole wheat bread crumbs
1 egg, beaten
2 tablespoons Worcestershire sauce
Salt and pepper to taste

Meal Prep
1) Preheat oven to 350°. Over medium heat, sauté onions in olive oil until translucent, approximately 5 minutes.

2) Add garlic and cook for an additional 2-3 minutes. Set aside and let cool to room temperature.

3) In a bowl combine ground turkey, parsley, tomato paste, bread crumbs, egg, Worcestershire sauce, salt, pepper, and onions. Mix well and place in a non-stick loaf pan. Bake for 45-50 minutes or until internal temperature reads 160°.

Pork Tenderloin With Spicy Red Pepper Sauce†

Makes about 5-6 servings

What You'll Need
2 pound loin of pork, boneless roast
1 tablespoon olive oil
Salt and pepper to taste
½ cup white wine

2 red peppers, roasted
2 cloves garlic
¼ cup low sodium chicken stock
1½ teaspoons red wine vinegar
Salt and pepper to taste
Pinch cayenne
Pinch red pepper flake
1 tablespoon extra virgin olive oil

Meal Prep
1) Preheat oven to 350° F. Rub the pork loin with olive oil and season with salt and pepper. Sear loin in a large sauté pan over medium high heat. Place tenderloin in roasting pan and cover with half of the wine. Cook at 350° for 1 hour, basting several times adding a little of the leftover wine each time you baste.

2) Roast peppers directly over gas stove until charred on all sides. Place peppers immediately into a brown bag and seal for 5 minutes.

3) Remove peppers, peel off charred skin and remove seeds. In a blender combine cooked peppers, garlic, chicken stock, vinegar, salt, pepper, cayenne, and red pepper flakes. Stream in olive oil until thoroughly pureed.

4) Warm sauce over medium heat for 2-3 minutes. Slice pork tenderloin and serve with red pepper sauce.

*One note: Add a small amount of cayenne pepper and red pepper flakes during Step 3. When the sauce is finished, taste it, and if you'd like it a bit more spicy, you can always stir in more cayenne and red pepper once the sauce is made.

Sweet Potato Latkas†
Makes 10 servings (2 latkas per serving)

What You'll Need
1 pound of sweet potatoes, peeled and grated
2 scallions (aka green onions), finely chopped
½ cup of whole wheat flour
2 eggs, lightly beaten
1 teaspoon salt
½ teaspoon pepper
¾ cup of vegetable oil

Meal Prep
1) Mix potatoes, scallions, flour, eggs, salt, and pepper.

2) In a large frying pan, heat oil on medium high heat for 5 minutes.

3) Form sweet potato mixture into 10 patties, ¼ inch thick and about the size of a pancake.

4) Cook latkas in oil until golden brown, about 2 minutes on each side. Place latkas on a paper towel and gently pat on top with an additional paper towel to remove excess oil.

Chapter #6
Eating Out

Americans are eating out much more than they used to. Our busy schedules have dramatically reduced the amount of time that we have to shop and prepare home cooked meals. This is a huge problem, and has much to do with the shocking increases in overweight and obesity over the past 30 years. In this chapter, we'll cover some of the problems with eating out, and give you some real world tips to help you do it in a way that won't sabotage your weight loss goals.

Why Eating Out Is A Problem

One thing that you always need to keep in mind about restaurants is that they are businesses. Like all businesses, their primary objective is to make money. They do not have your health as their main goal. They are not thinking about your weight loss goals. Their main objective is getting you back in their restaurant again and again and again.

While I was getting my PhD at Harvard, I attended a lecture that forever changed the way that I looked at eating out, and food companies in general. The speaker was the head nutrition researcher for a large food company that had an impressive line of both beverage and food items. He went on to mention that every time that their sales dropped, they would add more sugar, salt, or fat to their products, and sales would rise right back up.

They are not alone in this practice. Restaurants know how to addict you to their food, and they have become masters at it. They don't just want you to have a good meal and say, "That tasted awesome, I want to come back here sometime". They want you back tomorrow and the next day. They are pretty good at this too. Restaurant chains and food companies spend millions of dollars per year on researching the right combination of fat, salt, and sugar to addict you to their food.

I don't mean to blast away at restaurants and food companies here. There is room for just about every food in moderation, and at the end of the day, nobody forces us to make poor food choices; it is up to us. However, understanding that you are often getting a lot more junk in your restaurant food than you suspect is really important. In general, restaurant food has an over abundance of:

1) Calories
2) Fat
3) Saturated Fat
4) Sugar
5) Salt

Here are a few tips to help guide you through the treacherous waters of dining out:

1) *Don't eat out as much as you do right now.* It sounds simple. It is simple. Eat out less. When you shop and prepare your own food, you are in complete control of what you are eating. In restaurants, you are hopelessly out of control and at the mercy of the chef. Remember, the chef's primary goal is to improve the taste of the dish, not improve your health. Do your grocery shopping once a week, and get enough food to prepare the lion's share of your meals at home. It may be an obvious strategy, but it is the most important one.

2) *Use your splurge meals strategically.* You have two meals a week to go off the plan and eat whatever you want (except for sugar). If you know you'll be eating out, use one of these splurge meals, and you won't have to worry about being perfect. Splurge meals are great when you can't control your food 100%. Saving them for when you eat out is a great strategy to stay on top of your game.

3) *Do some online menu research.* Almost all restaurants now have their menus online. Check them out. Come up with a list of restaurants in your area where you can eat clean, and another list for the "splurge only" spots. In Boston, I know a bunch of local restaurants where I can always find great options when

I want to eat healthy. There are also restaurants that I know are great for splurge meals. Where I go depends on what I'm doing with my diet that night.

4) *Don't be afraid to ask for what you want.* Most restaurants are more than happy to substitute menu items if you ask. When I'm at a restaurant that I'm not too familiar with, I'll scan all the menu selections to see what side dishes are available. I recently was at a restaurant that had a healthy grilled fish dish that came with a potato side. I noticed that a steak dish came with sautéed spinach. I ordered the fish, but asked to substitute the spinach for the potato. The chef was more than happy to do so.

5) *Some specific guidelines:*
    *Start with a protein. Virtually any restaurant will have a variety of proteins to choose from. Look for options that don't have a lot of sauces, such as grilled chicken, fish, lean steak, or seafood.

    *Shoot for vegetables for your carbs. This includes salads, sautéed vegetables or sweet potatoes. If the restaurant offers whole grains like brown rice or quinoa, feel free to add one of these as well.

    *Use healthy vegetable oils to round out your fat serving. Ask for olive oil and vinegar on the side when ordering a salad, or ask that your vegetables be sautéed in olive or canola oil.

*Limit sauces and dressings that are creamy or sweet. Always get your sauce or dressing on the side, and put a reasonable amount on your dish. A good guideline is to put half of what they give you on your food.

*When the server brings bread, kindly refuse it. If service is on the slow side and you're hungry, seeing warm bread and butter may be too much for you!

*If possible, substitute brown rice for white rice. Many restaurants can now accommodate this request.

*If a dish comes with pasta, white rice, or potatoes, ask for sautéed vegetables or a side salad instead.

*In general, stay away from prepared salad dressings. They are usually too high in saturated fat and/or sugar. Instead, ask for olive oil and vinegar on the side. This way you can control your fat portion completely.

6) *Be an early bird.* Eating out and eating late seem to go hand in hand. This is a 1–2 punch combination to your waistline that is difficult to defend. Do your best to make reservations as early as possible. Remember that you need to be done eating by 8:00 PM. When you absolutely can't control the time of your reservation (at a business meeting, for example), eat before you go and

get a small salad or bowl of soup for your entrée. I've had clients in the past successfully use this strategy.

Chapter #7
Travel

Traveling presents some unique challenges for those trying to lose weight. Here are some of the major issues:

1) We are in far less control of our food.
2) It is more difficult to exercise.
3) We tend to drink more alcohol.
4) Our sleep is often disrupted.
5) A "vacation mentality" lends to a more carefree attitude regarding our diet and exercise.
6) We eat out every meal. This has a negative impact on our calorie, fat, salt, and sugar intake.

I think of travel as falling into two separate categories. The first is vacation travel. This type of travel happens for most of us only once a year, and will last for about a week on average. The second type of travel is more frequent work related travel. For a number of my clients, work related travel amounts to 50% of the year. Each type of travel requires a distinct strategy, and therefore, we will deal with each separately.

Vacation

Here are some tips to help you deal with vacation travel. Once again, this type of travel is of short duration and happens infrequently, usually only once a year for most of us.

1) *Adjust Your Goals.* Here's a statement that may surprise you: you are not going to lose weight on vacation so don't even try to! Your goal for vacation is weight maintenance, but in all likelihood, you'll gain a few pounds. If you go away for only one week a year, I expect and even want you to have some fun! You'll probably eat a bit more and drink a bit more, and the truth of the matter is that you should, it's your vacation!

Go away with the attitude that you'll try to maintain your weight or even gain a pound or two. Any weight that you add will come off quickly once you get back and resume your healthy lifestyle. The truth of the matter is that you simply can't do that much damage in one week, especially if you follow these tips.

2) *Maintain Your Exercise To Minimize The Damage.* I don't recommend cutting back on your exercise during vacation. Get your daily cardio, and hit the weights a few times during the week. It should be easier to find time to exercise on vacation than any

other time of the year. In fact, when I go away, exercise is really the only thing on my to do list. I will not even think about booking a trip to a hotel or resort without gym facilities.

3) *Eat Conservatively For Breakfast And Lunch, Splurge A Bit On Dinner.* Eat a healthy breakfast and lunch as you normally would at home. Feel free to splurge a bit on dinner. This ensures that you will be eating sensibly most of the time, but will allow you to eat for fun each day of your vacation as well.

4) *Stay Away From Sugar, Even On Your Vacation.* Sugar is unique in its ability to completely derail your diet. I've seen it hundreds of times. If you have sugar even once, you start to want it again. Then you have it again, and want it some more. After a few days of this, other refined carbs like bread, pasta, white rice, and potatoes become irresistible to you.

The solution is to just stay away from sugar, even on vacation. Feel free to enjoy a sugar free dessert if it is available. I know that most cruise ships now serve a variety of sugar free desserts. In time, I'm confident we'll see more and more sugar free offerings at restaurants and resorts. However, if you don't think they will be available, bring some sugar free cookies along with you on vacation and eat them for dessert. Avoid sugar at all times and at all costs.

5) Prepare For Increased Cravings When You Return Home From Your Vacation. After splurging a bit more on your vacation, carb cravings will likely return with a vengeance. Prepare for them mentally. Also prepare for them by having all of your healthy foods stocked and ready as soon as you get back. A trip to the grocery store immediately upon your return is a necessity. After a few days you should be fine, particularly if you avoided sugar.

More Frequent Work Related Travel

If you travel often for work, a different strategy is necessary. You cannot allow yourself to get into a situation where you blow off your diet and exercise every time you are on a trip. You've got to learn to function on the road as you would at home. This is difficult, but not impossible. It is all about preparation, planning ahead, and keeping your diet and exercise goals a priority when you are away. Following are a few tips for the more frequent business traveler.

1) *If At All Possible, Travel Less.* If you are at all able to control your travel schedule, do everything you can to minimize the number of trips or the length of your trips. I do understand that this is not a possibility for a great number of business travelers. However, if you are self-employed or in control of your travel schedule, this is a great place to start.

2) *Keep Exercise On Your Schedule While Away.* Just because you are away for a few days doesn't mean that you can blow off your exercise. Book a hotel with a gym and use it. Over the years, I've learned that more often than not, business dinners go hand in hand with business travel. Therefore, your best bet is to wake up early and get your exercise in before your first meeting. If you absolutely can't find time to exercise during your trip, do more cardio before you leave and after you get back to make up the minutes so you still hit your weekly goal.

3) *Use Your Splurge Meals Strategically.* You have two meals a week to eat whatever you want. If you save them both for your business trip, you'll be OK if you can't control your food.

4) *Bring Some Food Along With You.* It's a great idea to bring some non-perishable food items along with you when you travel for a quick and healthy meal on the go. This works especially well for breakfast and lunch. For example, a low fat mozzarella cheese stick, an apple, and some nuts can be a quick breakfast that will keep your blood sugar stable. Likewise, a tuna pouch, some nuts, and fruit make for a great lunch. All of these items travel well, can be eaten on the go (even in an airplane), and don't need to be refrigerated. Packing a few of these meals will help you avoid the carb crazy continental breakfasts at hotels or a fast food lunch.

When I was getting my second Masters degree, the program was several hours away from my home and lasted all day Saturday and all day Sunday, one weekend a month. I spent Saturday night at a hotel. I would be away for two lunches, one breakfast and one dinner. Here was my strategy:

1) Bring breakfast for Sunday.

2) Bring lunch for Saturday and Sunday.

3) Use a splurge meal for Saturday night and eat out.

I'd leave that weekend eating exactly the way I wanted to, because I took the time to really plan ahead my meals and bring the right food with me on my trip.

5) *When Eating Out, Follow The Strategies Listed In The Last Chapter.* In the last chapter, we went over some great strategies to help you stay on course while eating at restaurants. Get to know these strategies, and bring them on the road with you when traveling!

Chapter #8
The Sugar Free Life

As previously mentioned, sugar is an absolute disaster for those trying to lose weight and improve their health. It is highly addictive. The more you eat it, the more you want it. Sugar increases hunger and food cravings. It has also been associated with a number of chronic diseases. The best way to handle sugar is to eliminate it from your diet. Even tiny amounts of sugar can cause tremendous cravings in most people. It seems strange saying this, but it is far easier to give up sugar 100% than to give it up 75%.

The overwhelming majority of my clients that have hit their goal weight have sworn off sugar. I, personally, have not touched sugar for over 15 years. I know this sounds intimidating. The idea of giving up sugar initially terrified me.

However, it is not nearly as difficult as you might think. 1) After two weeks without sugar, if you are following this blood sugar stabilizing diet, your cravings for it virtually disappear. I've learned that cravings for sugar are much more physiological than psychological. Get it out of your diet, get through two weeks of withdrawal, and your desire for sugar will diminish to a level you never thought possible. 2) Sugar free versions of just about every dessert imaginable are now widely available.

Many of my clients are uncomfortable with the idea of non-nutritive sweeteners at first. There are a lot of myths about them and there are a few problems with them as well. In this chapter, we'll go over everything you need to know about non-nutritive sweeteners, and list the best sugar free items out there and how to get them.

Artificial Sweeteners (AKA Non-nutritive Sweeteners)

Artificial sweeteners have been the subject of controversy since their inception in 1879. A variety of myths and misconceptions concerning their health effects have been swirling around for decades. Let's lay out the facts. Non-nutritive sweeteners are food additives that provide a sweet taste without providing caloric energy. The FDA has approved the use of five non-nutritive sweeteners.

1) Aspartame: found in Equal and Nutrasweet
2) Acesulfame K: found in Sunett and Sweet One
3) Saccharin: found in Sweet 'N Low
4) Sucralose: found in Splenda
5) Neotame: does not have any brand names

Are Artificial Sweeteners Safe?

Despite popular belief, the FDA approved non-nutritive sweeteners are extremely well tested for safety. These sweeteners have been tested at levels of consumption so high that a person could never attain them in every day life, yet still produced no negative effects on health. I recently read a review paper on all of the non-nutritive sweeteners and the summary finding was that they were not associated with any negative health outcomes. After reviewing the literature, I can say with confidence that occasional use of these additives will not cause brain tumors, stroke, seizures, Alzheimer's disease, or any of the other maladies that people associate with them.

Does This Mean We Can Use Them All The Time?

This is where it gets a little bit tricky. I do not recommend the use of non-nutritive sweeteners on an everyday basis. Although they won't cause serious health problems, there are two major issues with them:

Issue #1: Non nutritive sweeteners perpetuate cravings for sugar and refined carbohydrate foods.

Once you limit your intake of refined carbohydrate foods like white bread, white rice, pasta, potatoes, and sugar, you'll notice that you stop craving them. This is especially true if you give up these foods in the context of a stable blood sugar, as you will with *The Weight*

Loss Triad. If you are eating non-nutritive sweeteners on a daily basis, you'll never get over your cravings for refined carbohydrates. You will be hungry all the time. This is a problem because any diet that involves feelings of deprivation and hunger will not work long term.

Issue #2: The cephalic response.

The second problem with non-nutritive sweeteners gets a bit more technical. We humans have something called the cephalic response. If I was to put your favorite food in front of you, your eyes would see it, your nose would smell it, and your body will actually release digestive enzymes before you even put a bite into your mouth. Your body is anticipating consumption. This is very likely happening when you consume non-nutritive sweeteners. Your body thinks it is getting something sweet, so it releases insulin anyway. This is the exact situation that we are trying to avoid, since the resulting drop in blood sugar following an insulin surge will leave you ravenous.

In light of these two problems, I do not recommend non-nutritive sweeteners for everyday use. However, used occasionally, I believe that they are far less harmful than sugar. At the end of the day, I can't produce a single, well designed research paper that shows an association between occasional non-nutritive sweetener use and any chronic disease. On the other hand, I can produce dozens, if not hundreds of research papers that show an association between high glycemic load carbohydrates, such as sugar, and chronic diseases like heart disease, stroke, diabetes, certain cancers, and obesity.

Since you are allowed two splurge meals per week, this is the time you are permitted to dive into the world of non-nutritive sweeteners. Limiting non-nutritive sweetener consumption to these two meals gives you the best of both worlds. You can enjoy something sweet a couple of times per week to satisfy your cravings for dessert, but you can also ensure a stable blood sugar to keep food cravings from getting out of control.

What About Stevia?

Stevia is another non-nutritive sweetener that is produced from the leaves of a plant grown in Southern and Central America. While Stevia producers say it is safe, the FDA has not done its own evaluation just yet. The FDA initially agreed to the manufacturer's safety findings and has allowed it to be used in a variety of products. More recently, there have been some reports that Stevia may increase cancer risk, so the FDA is requiring more information on the safety of the sweetener. Personally, I feel that Stevia has not been tested enough for me to recommend it to my clients. I'd limit use until we learn more.

What About Sugar Alcohols?

Sugar alcohols are compounds that taste sweet like sugar, but are not as easily broken down and absorbed as table sugar. On food labels, they show up as xylitol, mannitol, erythritol, hydrogenated starch hydrolysates, and sorbitol. Sugar alcohols are found in nature in prunes and apricots. Sugar alcohols generally have 50-70% of the sweetness of sugar. They are cropping up in all sorts of sugar free items, particularly sugar free candy and ice cream. The only problem that I have seen regarding their safety is that they can have a laxative effect when consumed in large quantities because they are not completely absorbed. Therefore, start with small amounts of sugar alcohols and see how you react to them. It's easy to tell how much you are getting because the grams of sugar alcohol will be right on the food label under carbohydrates.

Sugar Free Versus No Sugar Added

One more note, dairy products have a naturally occurring sugar called lactose. This is a low glycemic sugar that is easy on the blood sugar and not a problem. However, because of this, dairy products like ice cream won't say sugar free on the package but will say "No Sugar Added". For the most part, these two terms are interchangeable.

The Best Sugar Free Products And Where To Get Them

Over the years, and with help from my clients, I have discovered some really good sugar free products to enjoy on splurge meals. Here's a list of the best of the best. Some are really easy to find, some you'll have to order online. Remember—don't go overboard with the sugar free stuff. You can only have these sugar free treats twice per week with your splurge meals.

Edy's No Sugar Added Ice Cream: Most grocery store chains carry this in their freezer section. It comes in a bunch of great flavors, including Triple Chocolate, Mint Chip, Fudge Tracks, Neapolitan, and Vanilla. Turkey Hill, Blue Bunny, and Breyer's also make no sugar added ice cream that is really good.

Murray's Sugar Free Cookies: These are the best sugar free cookies that I've found by far. You can usually find these in your grocery store. If not, you can order them on Amazon.com. They have an amazing selection, including: Chocolate Chip, Oatmeal, Peanut Butter, Fudge Dipped Mint, Fudge Dipped Grahams, Sandwich Cookies, and more.

Klondike No Sugar Added Ice Cream Bars: These are outstanding and can usually be found in your grocery store's freezer section. They come in two varieties, Vanilla and Crunch. I strongly recommend the Crunch!

Stop And Shop Brand No Sugar Added Ice Cream Sandwiches: Exclusive to Stop And Shop super-markets. These are unbelievably good.

Hershey's Sugar Free Chocolates: These are usually available in the chain pharmacies like CVS, Rite Aid, and Walgreens. They come in Special Dark or Milk Chocolate. Stick with small quantities because these are very high in sugar alcohols which can have a laxative effect in sensitive individuals.

Reeses' Sugar Free Miniature Peanut Butter Cups: These can be found in pharmacies like CVS, Rite Aid, and Walgreens. They are very good. Stick with small quantities because they are high in sugar alcohols.

Sugar Free York Peppermint Patties: Also found in pharmacies. Also high in sugar alcohols, so limit amounts here.

Russell Stover Sugar Free Candy: You can find this amazing selection of candy in most pharmacies. They make Mint Patties, Crispy Caramel, Pecan Delights, Peanut Butter Crunch, Chocolate Coconut, Chocolate Covered Peanuts, and many more. Again, these are high in sugar alcohols so limit amounts. If you can't find these in stores, you can get them online at www.russellstover.com

Tastykake Sensables: These are truly amazing! They make cupcakes, coffee cakes, finger cakes, and cookie bars that are sugar free and taste great. You can find these in certain grocery chains, but they seem to be getting harder to find in stores. You can always get them online at www.netrition.com.

Sugar Free Oreos: Can be found at some grocery stores and online at www.netrition.com. These are delicious.

Voortman's Sugar Free Cookies: These are terrific. They come in great flavors like Chocolate Chip, Oatmeal, and Vanilla Wafers. You can usually find these in your supermarket cookie section.

Sugar Free Jello And Chocolate Pudding: Sugar free Jello and Chocolate Pudding can be found in just about any supermarket. A spoonful of Sugar Free Cool Whip on top takes this to a whole new level.

EAS Low Carb AdvantEdge Bars: These protein bars are sugar free and come in great flavors like Chocolate Chip Brownie and Chocolate Peanut Butter. These taste more like a candy bar than a protein bar. You can find these at GNC or order them by the box at vitamin-shoppe.com. Met-RX Protein Plus bars are similar to the EAS bars and taste just as good.

Pillsbury Sugar Free Brownie Mix: These come in Milk Chocolate and Chocolate Fudge flavors. They are really good and can be found in most supermarkets. Go easy with the portions here as these are quite high in sugar alcohols.

Pillsbury Sugar Free Cake Mix: This comes in Vanilla or Chocolate flavor and can be found in most grocery store bakery aisles. They also sell a sugar free frosting, but this is loaded with trans fat, so I would skip it and instead use....

Sweet 'N Low Sugar Free Frosting: This comes in Vanilla or Chocolate flavors. There is a very slight Sweet 'N Low aftertaste with this frosting, but overall it is very good. We make cupcakes with this frosting and the Pillsbury Sugar Free Cake Mix. You generally won't find the Sweet 'N Low frosting in stores but can get it online at www.edietshop.com.

Sugar Free Pancake Syrup: Great for a breakfast splurge of pancakes or French toast. Log Cabin makes one, and so does Cary's. Both taste great, in fact, I can't tell the difference between these and regular syrup. You can almost always find these in grocery stores. Many restaurants serving breakfast now carry these so don't be afraid to ask for them!

DaVinci Sugar Free Syrups: These are awesome if you like to make flavored Lattes. They come in a lot of great flavors like Caramel, Chocolate, French Vanilla, Hazel Nut, Irish Cream, and many more. You can find these online at www.davincigourmet.com.

Sugar Free Cool Whip: Great on fresh fruit or sugar free ice cream. You can find this in most any grocery store.

Swiss Miss No Sugar Added Hot Chocolate: Delicious and found in most grocery stores.

Smucker's Sugar Free Grape Jelly: Really good and found in most grocery stores. This is high in sugar alcohol, so go easy on portions with this one. You can also get these online at www.smuckers.com.

Smucker's Sugar Free Hot Fudge: Found in grocery stores or online at www.smuckers.com. Great on sugar free ice cream. Also comes in caramel flavor. High in sugar alcohols so go easy on the portions.

Cheesecake Factory Low Carb Cheesecake: This may be the best sugar free dessert that I have ever tried. Found at the Cheesecake Factory restaurants (they also do take out). It comes with sugar free whipped cream and strawberries. Make this a very occasional treat because it is very high in saturated fat and calories.

There you have it. These should hold you for a while! Remember, sugar free treats are only for your two splurge meals. The rest of the time you need to avoid non-nutritive sweeteners. The good news is that once your blood sugar stabilizes, you won't really even crave them.

Chapter #9
Shopping Guide

Eating healthy used to be completely normal and quite easy for us. While evolving, the right foods were readily available, and there was no such thing as junk food. My, how things have changed! The norm now is to eat unhealthy. Everywhere we go: restaurants, ball games, the movies, coffee shops, airports, rest stops, etc, there are tons of unhealthy food choices and very few healthy ones.

Your home has to become your oasis for healthy eating. This means doing your own grocery shopping, and cooking your meals the vast majority of the time. Therefore, I thought it might be helpful to list out the top 15 food items to always keep in your pantry or refrigerator. If you have these tried and true, nutrient packed foods ready to go, you are never more than a few minutes away from a healthy, blood sugar stabilizing meal.

#1 Vegetables: Variety is the key here, and the more the merrier. Include vegetables for salads, sweet potatoes, broccoli, cauliflower, spinach, and on and on.

#2 Fruits: Again, variety is the key. Make sure to get a bunch of fruits that travel well, such as apples and pears. You can throw these in a backpack or purse and they are always ready for you no matter what your day brings.

#3 Nuts: An excellent source of healthy fat that travels well.

#4 Nut Butters: Peanut butter, almond butter, cashew butter, macadamia nut butter, pistachio butter. They are all really good.

#5 Olive Oil: Great for salad dressing and to sauté vegetables.

#6 Old Fashioned Slow Cooked Oatmeal: A nice lower glycemic whole grain packed with fiber. Don't get instant or quick cooking as these are higher glycemic. Focus on the "Old Fashioned" slow cooking variety.

#7 Black Beans: Great in a salad or even on their own. These are a very good source of low glycemic carbohydrate and vegetable protein loaded with fiber, vitamins, and minerals. Try to find a low sodium version.

#8 Quinoa: An awesome whole grain that is high in fiber and protein. This is relatively new here in America but can be found in most grocery stores. We cook ours in low sodium chicken broth, and it is a great dinner side dish.

#9 Tuna Pouches: These are relatively new. They are tuna fish in a pouch that you simply tear open and eat. You don't need to drain this tuna or use a can opener. Highly portable, these are great on the road or even on an airplane.

#10 Chicken Breast: Buy in bulk at Costco or BJ's and keep in your freezer. When combined with the George Foreman Grill, you've got a beautifully grilled chicken breast in about 6 minutes.

#11 Eggs: An excellent source of both fat and protein. They take about 5 minutes to prepare when cooking them and even less if you hard boil them ahead of time and have them ready to go.

#12 Olivio or Smart Balance: These are butter substitutes made from olive and canola oil. You can use these any time you'd use butter. They taste really good and are so much better for you than butter.

#13 Brown Rice: A great lower glycemic whole grain that is a good source of cereal fiber. Make sure you get

the slow cooked variety and not instant or quick cooking as these are higher glycemic.

#14 Sliced Turkey Breast: A low fat, convenient source of protein. Try to get it freshly sliced off a bird and not the pre-packaged variety that is filled with nitrates and preservatives.

#15 Frozen Shrimp: A delicious source of protein that is surprisingly reasonable when bought frozen in bulk at Costco or BJ's.

Also By Dr. Thomas L. Halton:

The Weight Loss Triad
A Comprehensive Guide To Lasting Weight Loss

Maximize Your Health
The Top Ten Research Proven Strategies To
Reduce Your Risk Of Chronic Disease

If you need more guidance, Dr. Halton is
available for phone consultations. Learn more at:
www.drtomhalton.com/phone

Dr. Halton also publishes a free e-newsletter.
Learn more and sign-up at:
www.drtomhalton.com/newsletter

Made in the USA
Middletown, DE
30 July 2019